FOREWORD BY REV. DR. AHRIANA PLATTEN

STORIES, TOOLS + COMMUNITY FOR

healing
—curious
humans

I0458982

NATALIE V. PETERSEN

FEATURING: LISA BOATE • SUE BRUCKNER • SHARON CASSIDY
LAURIE S. COSSAR • KIM LOUISE EDEN • AMANDA FUEL
TINA GREEN • R. SCOTT HOLMES • LEAH JOHNSON
DR. TIFFANY McBRIDE • FALYN HUNTER MORNINGSTAR
IAN MORRIS • PATTY NAGLE • RUBY RAJA
MADISEN ROSE • SUSAN SCHILLER • NANCY TERRY
MANDY WEBB HANCOCK • SILEN WELLINGTON

FOREWORD BY REV. DR. AHRIANA PLATTEN

STORIES, TOOLS + COMMUNITY FOR
healing –curious humans

NATALIE V. PETERSEN

FEATURING: LISA BOATE • SUE BRUCKNER • SHARON CASSIDY
LAURIE S. COSSAR • KIM LOUISE EDEN • AMANDA FUEL
TINA GREEN • R. SCOTT HOLMES • LEAH JOHNSON
DR. TIFFANY McBRIDE • FALYN HUNTER MORNINGSTAR
IAN MORRIS • PATTY NAGLE • RUBY RAJA
MADISEN ROSE • SUSAN SCHILLER • NANCY TERRY
MANDY WEBB HANCOCK • SILEN WELLINGTON

ADVANCE PRAISE FOR
HEALING-CURIOUS HUMANS

"Like a giant door swinging wide open, *Healing-Curious Humans* is an invitation to sit with an old friend who knows your soul. She's offered a cup of tea and says, "It's time." Time to go inward, to explore, to remember you're not lost—you're being called. Honest, broken, open, fearless, triumphant! This book helps us honor who we've been and who we're becoming. What a beautiful companion for anyone ready to begin again and again and again!"

~ Stephanie Urbina Jones and Jeremy Pajer,
Co-Founders, Freedom Folk and Soul

"*Healing-Curious Humans* held me tightly in its embrace as the authors shared intense stories of how they survived some of the most terrifying times in their lives. Their courage and strength shine like a bright beacon, beckoning the reader forward to join their journeys to wellness. The tools provided add much-needed support for others struggling to escape abuse. I am overcome with gratitude for this book."

~ Dr. Ruth Souther, Founder of Vega's Path Priestess Process

"*Healing-Curious Humans* doesn't just tell stories; it offers tools for readers to explore their own curiosity. It's intimate, brave, and aligned with the kind of impact we hope to foster in Hey Birdie Flocks. We recommend this book to anyone wanting to reconnect with awe, discover tools for self-exploration, and witness the power of curiosity in action. *Healing-Curious Humans* is a gift of insight and inspiration, and it resonates deeply with our own mission."

~ Jessica Lindsley and Heather Bahlmann, Founders, Hey Birdie

Dedication

This one's for Me.

The Me who didn't quit, even when the path disappeared.

The Me who kept asking questions even when no one was answering.

The Me who got curious instead of bitter, soft instead of shut down.

The Me who chose to live. Again and again.

I wrote this book for her. To honor her.

Me.

Because for so long, I didn't believe she was worth honoring.

As you hold this book in your hands,

perhaps part of you is ready to let go of, finally, the same.

As you read, join me in making this dedication to the Me in You.

Let us speak it to our Past Self.

Let us offer it to our Now Self.

Let us whisper it to the version of each one of us

who is just beginning.

I am the reason I made it here.

That deserves to be named.

You are the reason you made it here.

Let us name that together, too.

This book is dedicated to Me.

And as a gift from my heart to yours,

It is, with unconditional love, dedicated to *You*.

DISCLAIMER

This book is designed to provide competent, reliable, and educational information on mind, body, and spiritual health and wellness, as well as other related subject matter. However, it is sold with the understanding that the authors and publisher specifically disclaim all responsibility for any liability, loss, or risk, personal or otherwise, incurred as a consequence, directly or indirectly, of the use and application of any of the contents of this publication.

In order to maintain the anonymity of others, the names and identifying characteristics of some people, places, and organizations described in this book have been changed.

This publication contains content that may be potentially triggering or disturbing. Individuals who are sensitive to certain themes are advised to exercise caution while reading.

The opinions, ideas, and recommendations contained in this publication do not necessarily represent those of the publisher. The use of any information provided in this book is solely at your own risk.

Our authors represent cultures worldwide, and as such, there may be differences in language and expressions. As a global publisher, we have made the conscious choice not to edit these nuances, so each chapter is authentic and in its author's words.

Know that the experts here have shared their tools, practices, and knowledge with you with a sincere and generous intent to assist you on your personal journey. Please contact them with any questions you may have about the techniques or information they provided. They will be happy to assist you further and be an ongoing resource for your success!

Foreword

Rev. Dr. Ahriana Platten

Curiosity isn't a soft skill; it's the soul's first act of defiance against fear.

Not the kind of curiosity that makes you check your ex's social media at midnight or Google your headache until you're convinced you have something that hasn't been discovered yet. I'm talking about *sacred curiosity*. The kind that leans in when life gets messy. The kind that whispers *there's something here for you*, even when you just want to scroll past it, binge on Oreos, or run.

Real curiosity isn't aimless or shallow. It's not confusion masquerading as openness. It's the soul's way of tugging on your sleeve and saying, *Pay attention*. And maybe even more than that, *Be brave enough to stay with what you find*.

We think of it as childlike because it flows easily when we're young, but it's when we allow curiosity to accompany our grown-up life that we find awe in the adventure our experiences offer us.

So why did we forsake curiosity in the first place? Because we've been warned, haven't we? About curiosity? "Curiosity killed the cat." "Don't open that box, Pandora." "Don't go digging into things you don't understand." What if you uncover something you can't fix? What if the truth requires change? What if you lose control?

Here's the uncomfortable secret: *you were never in control.*

Curiosity leads to transformation. It's like gravity. You don't have to understand how it works. You just have to know that it does, and that resisting it only makes the landing harder.

That's where this book comes in.

It doesn't claim to have every answer. It doesn't wrap things in pretty bows or pretend healing is linear. Instead, it invites you into a more meaningful kind of dialogue. The kind where your body, your spirit, and your intuition get to speak. It asks you to meet yourself with wonder instead of wariness. To explore instead of escape. To breathe instead of brace.

Healing isn't something you conquer. It's something you befriend. And curiosity is how you get introduced.

When we stop rushing to fix what we don't yet understand, something beautiful begins to unfold. Judgment quiets. The edges soften. We begin to see the intelligence in our emotions, the wisdom in our wounds, and the messages in our mess.

Stories, Tools + Community for Healing-Curious Humans is a compilation of stories by my dear friend Natalie Petersen and a brilliant cohort of author experts. It teaches us how to hold a moment of curiosity open. How to live inside the question instead of scrambling for the exit, and to honor the unknown with just enough reverence and just enough humor to keep us grounded when what we discover feels like it might swallow us whole.

This book isn't a roadmap. It's more like a candle. You carry it into the darker rooms of your inner world. You notice what's there. You listen. And slowly, darkness shifts to illumination.

So, if you've arrived here with questions, and maybe with hope, or maybe with a little bit of both…welcome. Let this book accompany you as you wander through the landscapes of your own healing. Let it challenge your old assumptions, spark your creativity, and give you permission to stay curious, even when it's uncomfortable.

Because beneath all the striving and the fear, something wise in you already knows curiosity is not a threat.

It's the way home.

May you read slowly.

May you breathe deeply.

May you trust your unfolding.

Dr. Ahriana Platten
Bestselling Author of *Rites and Rituals* and *The Changing Story*

Table of Contents

Introduction

Once upon a time, there was a human.

She was born curious, so damn curious.

She was the kind of child who tilted her head at birds when they spoke,

Who asked too many questions at dinner,

And wondered what made the moon

Follow her home only on certain nights.

But along the way—slowly, subtly—

Her curiosity got smooshed.

Scolded. Dismissed.

Wrapped in sticky, sludgy shame and labeled "too much."

So, she stopped asking.

She didn't stop *wondering*, no.

But she stuffed her questions deep into invisible pockets.

And with each unasked question,

Her vibrant, bright light dimmed just a bit more.

She felt crummy.

High points were sunny, sure.

But the low points?

They were heavy and hollow,

With a kind of sadness that didn't always have a name,

And one she often wasn't sure would let go.

She kept a secret list.

Scrawled in her mind,

Scribbled in the corners of her heart,

A list of questions she'd ask if she ever got brave enough.

Why do I feel like too much and not enough at the same time?

What if I stopped pretending I was okay?

Who am I without all this performing?

Is there still time for me to become who I am meant to be?

The list stayed with her, quietly waiting.

And so did the ache.

And then, one ordinary day,

After one too many polite smiles, and

One too many swallowed truths,

She cracked open.

Not with drama or fireworks.

Not with some grand awakening.

Just…a sigh.

A whisper, from the floor of her basement this time, not the bathroom.

A moment of, *"What if I asked just one question?"*

So, she grabbed her courage and a wad of tissue, and she did it.

She asked a question.

And the world didn't end.

In fact, something flickered back on inside her,

Like the just-faint strobe of a forgotten lightbulb.

Curiosity.

The innocent, eager kind.

She giggled.

And then, something different.

Warmer. Firmer.

Grown-ass curiosity.

Seasoned. Tender. Fierce as Hell.

And in that moment,

Just a few baby steps past the giggle,

She began again.

With a tiny step, a shaky voice, and a gigantic heart.

She asked, and she listened.

She wept, and she wondered.

She began to feel the Earth beneath her feet, not just as ground,
but as kin.

The sky above her, not just weather, but a witness.

The fire in her belly wasn't discomfort; it was direction.

And water.

Sacred water.

Quench this burst of her thirst!

She didn't find all the answers. She didn't need to.

She was remembering something deeper:

Healing is not about fixing.

It's about *returning*.

Melting into the never-never land of her being,

She blipped, flinched, covered her eyes, and squeaked,

"Wait! Is this just *me*?"

Eek! She peeked, and she could see.

It *wasn't* just her.

There were so many of us—walking wounded, quiet rebels,
secret seekers—

Waiting behind the curtains of our own conditioning.

Trained to stay small, stay polite, stay in line.

And always with something stirrrrrrrrrring inside.

Listen!

She did. She is.

She's me.

Pssssst! Pssssssssssssst!

I hear you! Yes, you!

Come out from behind the curtains.

Come into the light of your own knowing.

Question the unconscious notions of how the world works.

Dismantle the beliefs you didn't choose.

Let your heart, not your fear, lead your next chapter.

Open your eyes, your heart, your mind.

To the astonishing, bone-deep wonder of our existence.

We are sharing the same air, you and I.

We are sharing the same sun.

We are sharing the same moon, stars, and ground
beneath our primitive feet.

We are *already connected.*

Connected, we lay down judgment.

Connected, we lay down the exhausting need to get it right.

Connected, we let go of the shame that keeps any one of us
from trying at all.

And, instead, connected, we rise.

In the name of curiosity, in the name of compassion,

And at the very core of our spirit,

We understand: **LOVE**.

Because what is *healing*, really?

I can't define that for you, c'mon now.

Only *you* know what it means in your divine body, in your story, in your life.

Perhaps healing involves grieving for what you never had.

Maybe it's calling your power back.

Sometimes, it's actually falling apart—on purpose.

Or even coasting to a complete stop to let someone else drive for a minute while you recalibrate your route.

Gosh, friend, I don't know. But what I *can* tell you is this:

The thread running through every story in this book is not about performance, perfection, or prescription.

It's **unconditional love**.

Love for people across every walk of life.

Love for the land that holds us and the sky that humbles us.

Love for the fire inside every one of us that still burns.

Love for the wind that brushes the tender cheek like a mother, a lover, a reminder.

A cool, watery whisper that says:

You belong here.

Still. Always.

This book is not a manual.

It's not a fix-it plan.

It's a doorway.

It's a companion.

It's an irrevocable license to be curious,

And a gentle nudge toward *your own* definition of healing.

Whatever that looks like.

With whatever taste, volume, or color.

Whatever that needs to be in your sacred, still-beating heart.

Take what you need as you need it.

Perhaps share.

Leave the rest.

Etch your name in the memory stick before you go.

And if you're new to your journey and holding your own secret
list of questions?

Maybe now is the time to get curious yourself and ask just one.

You'll find a community here that'll be there to listen and support you.

And the way will illuminate, I promise.

Not brightly. Not all at once.

But enough.

Always enough.

I love you.

Natalie P.,
a fellow and forever Healing-Curious Human

CHAPTER 1

Breathing Air Into Every Episode

Your Unrehearsed, Raw Take Is Much Preferred

Natalie V. Petersen

Wonder is the beginning of all wisdom.

~ Socrates

MY STORY

I mean, seriously, Natalie?!

Who the hell are you to think anyone will want to read this?

That what you have to offer will even register on a radar, let alone change a life? That's rich, bitch.

They're hitting Like because they love you. It's the nice thing to do.

You all can hear your mind's voices, right?

Or maybe you're one of the lucky 30%-50% that don't have a constant dialogue running in your head. Dr. Russell T. Hurlburt, a professor of psychology at the University of Nevada, Las Vegas, and bestselling author of multiple books on the subject, will tell you there is silence in up to half of the population's minds!

Whoa. Mine's a nuthouse, and on any given day, any number of characters come out to play.

Like the current one sitting on my shoulder, the she-bully that squats rent-free in my mental space, heckling me in a tone that practically vibrates with judgment, with what she spends her time convincing me "they" are saying.

And to outwardly share deep thoughts and insight? Gross, Natalie. This is your bloody battle inside your head, not theirs!

She'll come at me from all directions.

There's no reason to spill this out there. Look around—people are already puking dysfunction everywhere. Do we need more? Does your story even matter amidst the shit? Like, reeeeeally?

Then Izzy buzzes in. She's the size of a gnat, and she zips and dips in and out of earshot. Her incessant voice flits in and out and around my head.

Button it up, buttercup. Fucking relax. Take some time off. Maybe d-e-t-o-x...?

Izzy has no mercy, and she moves at the pace of a hummingbird on steroids.

Wait, she'll buzz. *You're SOBER? Well then, therapy. Lots of therapy. Have you been to actual therapy? The kind that WORKS?*

And then, mid-tirade, she'll switch it up and lay on the gas.

While you're at it, figure out what you want to be when you fucking grow up. Geezus. Get out of your way, if you can, hag. People are tired of your same-ol' story! Fucking DO something. Find a passion, create a profession, make some profit, live happily ever after.

Ouch! Snap!

Mama Natalie, the martyr herself, has entered the room. Her's is a tone drunk with hidden meaning, laced with condescension and an undertone of rage. Her eyes suck air out of rooms and leave most feeling tiny.

Sit your happy little ass down. You have obligations before you do that, Missy. Lots of them, Ma-Ma.

Mama. Mother. Mom. Partner. Sister. Friend. Where do I begin...or could I end?

Yeah, mental health aware. That's me. That's the gist of this episode you've found me in. It took everything I had to get here because of the fucking headspace I've been in since Mother's Day.

I had such a beautiful day with my son. My heart is full of love and wonder when I'm with him. Our bond is real. Undeniable. When I'm in a slumpy space, I fill my heart with the awe I feel for him, the miracle of his life. He is a bright light in my world.

My son was born via surrogate—gestational surrogacy, actually—with a beautiful human named Darlene, who carried my baby as if he were her own.

She was on my mind all day, too, on Mother's Day. She's often on my mind. I think about her generosity as she walked beside me, hand-in-hand. I hope we can always be in touch.

I didn't think I deserved to be a mother, honestly—not after the abortion I had in my early 20s. When I got cervical cancer in my early 30s, I told the doctors without blinking: "Cut that shit out of me. It's cancer. I have a life to live."

What I didn't realize then was that I carried a silent sentence, that I buried shame and regret so deep, I didn't know it was still dictating what I thought I deserved.

When it came time for the radical hysterectomy, I went alone. My husband went hunting. Or was it work? Didn't matter. I wanted solitude. Punishment. Stillness.

I pushed my mother off until the end of my hospital stay. I needed the loneliness. I deserved it.

I made friends with the fringe night crew, laughed hard with a wonderfully gay nurse who built me a cheat board of foam and surgical tape to help me get out of bed without splitting stitches. I had surgery on Monday, was home by Friday, and threw a cocktail party by Sunday. Back to life, right?

I kept my ovaries—just in case. And to avoid early menopause. Not that I was planning for anything. I was still drinking, performing, and dangling off spreadsheets, numbing. Always numbing.

Then came a stirring of motherhood, and I wondered if I could finally patch my pain by outsourcing it. Buy the solution. Fix the ache—no help needed. Just go bigger.

I decided to have a child with my husband.

It was 2005-2006. We began the hunt for a surrogate. Our network and privilege made it easy. Nothing was covered by insurance—I wasn't having trouble conceiving, I was deemed infertile. It was a lovely word to swallow, along with so many other chemicals and pieces of advice, in the process.

We opted for the agency route. Too many hoops, otherwise. Too many rights, roles, and contractual oddities. I felt overwhelmed and vulnerable, and paying that much attention required me to be more clear-headed than I was in my adult life.

"Peace of mind," the agency said. We paid handsomely for it.

And it was peaceful. The people were terrific. I remember just a few of their names.

I used to tell a fucked-up joke here—because that's my shield, right? Shock and awe. Make you laugh before you look too closely.

It went like this:

I was drunk my entire pregnancy.

Bahhh dump.

While Darlene tended to our baby with her entire being, I drank. Hard. I doubled down. I numbed the fuck out.

I mean, c'mon now, there was now a neon-buzzing clock, flickering, and counting down 24/7 behind my eyes.

*Party now, because soon you'll be **Mom**, and you'll be perfect, sober, and glowing.*

This was The Great Reset.

I was gonna get sober and start living, like my parents never did for me. I'd show them, dammit.

We showed up for every appointment. I missed only one—the 3D ultrasound. When I saw the video, I knew: he was coming.

Our baby was due on Valentine's Day 2009.

My father died by suicide on Valentine's Day 1997.

I don't believe in coincidence.

Mental and spiritual illness have been part of my life longer than my memory. I recently found an old book. Tucked inside was a card in my childhood handwriting:

"Natalie's Library. Due date: 4/17."

On the back was a printed appointment card for Southwest Mental Health Clinic in Durango, Colorado.

I asked my mom. She vaguely remembered. She said it was probably hers, from when I was three. Postpartum. Breakdown. Depression.

Call it what you want. She struggled her whole life with medication, addiction, and with herself.

I don't remember her being gone, don't recall my mom leaving me because, she said, her own memory ignited, "I just couldn't stop crying. Days and days…"

But I remember the cigarette smoke. The haze. The hum of the box fan in our trailer window, and being the lucky one to flip it around to blow the cottonwood off the screen.

And I remember growing up *fast*. All of a sudden, being responsible for more than I thought was fair, I did not have the language to support my sacred body's acceleration.

But I also remember authentic joy. I remember my bright-eyed, blonde father behind the wheel of the '63 Olds, his tanned arm slung out the window, and my adventurous mom smiling in the passenger seat, her box perm still fresh. Red is the color of her handmade shorts.

I remember the corner of the hard, ribbed, and ripping edge of the big backseat that cut into my blonde-haired legs, as fast as I can feel the thrill to be heading into the magic of our natural playground. Like it was yesterday. There remain little dirt roads up into the hills where people go to hide, hunt, pray, and play all over that neck of the woods.

My brother and I began scrambling, readying ourselves as the car turned off Highway 160 onto the gravel road called First Notch, into the U.S. National Forest just outside my one-flashing-light hometown, Bayfield.

This scenario was our absolute favorite: the feeling of all four wheels leaving the pavement, the sound of back doors opening, and my brother and I clad in my mom's handstitched love scrambling aboard while the car rolled in neutral, my dad chuckling like his dad.

We hooked our fingers around the edge of the metal by the windshield, legs spread wide for leverage, thrilled to be exactly where we were for the adventure ahead.

"There's so much to explore up the road, get on!" We heard my parents smiling and laughing at us.

My dad leaned out the window, and my mom tapped the dashboard like she did. Not too hard, for hers was a quiet rebellion.

Our family binoculars around one lucky fool's neck, and everyone else assigned to pick and carry our treasures, we had snakes and horny toads, yarrow and wild acorns, and Rocky Mountain Columbine to admire.

We had tracks and arrowheads, topography and geography, birds, bears, and elk. Our compass? The sun, and landmarks like quirky little aspen groves and cool carvings we'd leave for other seekers. We monitored weather and were elated at possible rainstorms ahead.

Or the blessed breeze and the cool shade of a passing cloud on a hot, high-altitude day, a family nap, the four of us, in a big field under a lone pine tree with a Swallowtail or a lost cub as company.

The possibilities with my wild-spirited parents were simply endless.

In the mountains, we were free. Wild. Happy. Ourselves.

When the drinking started again, I was in high school. I'd already been experimenting with weed, acid, and mushrooms since I was thirteen. My parents had their addictions, which they held at bay since I was a baby. I had a running head-start on mine.

My father was a Christian, sometimes a minister, a farrier, a poet, and a small engine repairman.

My mom was a dutiful wife. She was fragile. As polished as she could stand. An English-degreed, wildly creative, posture-corrector and soul-preneur with what always felt like secrets. She believed in her place—beneath.

My mom tried to end her life more than once and in many ways. There was a significant period when I had to establish considerable boundaries between us to protect my heart and my son.

Now both parents are passed, and I'm a beautiful mess of holy and horrific memories-made-present-tense magic.

For too long, however, I let the tragedies play on repeat—like a greatest hits album for pain.

"Waaahhh-naaa-naa-NEEEOWWW!"

Think: epic face-melting air guitar solo, my mohawk on point, stage lights blinding.

Wait. Surprise!

My son came ten days early. We had a check-in with Darlene, and boom—delivery was happening the next day.

I panicked. Went out straightaway. Got drunk. Showed up the next morning still buzzing with fear and wine and shame. And brandishing a brand new video camera with a dead battery.

I didn't carry him. Darlene delivered him.

And I held her hand when he arrived.

Darlene was well-tended in recovery, but they didn't have a room for us intended parents. We met him in a converted NICU closet. He was tiny. Glossy-eyed. Without a name, because we just weren't sure yet.

And I breastfed him.

That was our first soul-connection earthside. And I knew. I knew I wanted to be someone he could count on.

But those early years were volatile, and there are days when that rebreaks a bit of my heart.

Like generations before him, my son has memories of experiences his wounded parents can't undo.

Raging perfectionism and fawning are particular aspects of my past that continue to elude me on occasion, but drinking was how I coped with it all. With emptiness. With anxiety. With not knowing how to be *me* without the high.

As a new mom, my nickname was Happy Hour.

By the end, it was straight vodka in mason jars. No ice. Extra shame.

I got sober nearly seven years ago, as of the publication of this chapter. Not because I hit a rock bottom, but because I slammed into something more complex.

Myself.

The surround sound message was deafening and brought me to my knees in the shiny, new, spacious shower of Divorced Natalie's condo.

GET YOUR FUCKING SHIT TOGETHER, WOMAN. Your son is watching, I heard pipe through the shower head and reverberate in every drop of water hitting my fully exposed body.

And he was.

I told him the truth:

"I choose love. Our love. Over the bottle."

My son believed me because I meant it.

Even now, miles down the road, I still have days on the bathroom floor.

But I'm here. And I'm free.

I feel young. Wild. Brand new.

And I can hear my dad say, "It's an adventure, Nut!" as I greet each day.

At 50, I'm just getting started. I want it all—the pain, the joy, the questions, the stretch, the marks.

Life is a wild ride of valleys and peaks and algorithmic despair. Can you feel me?

And still—I choose it. Click, click, click on the algorithm of love.

We can numb it all out. Scroll it down. Drink it, reflect it, project it, binge it away.

But this work—the work of *being*—isn't going anywhere.

So instead of abandoning yourself again, dear, new friend of mine, what if you just got curious with me?

I know, I know, this was all about me. Most folks' stories are, huh? Life is curious and fantastic like that. We reflect others' lives through stories of our own.

Indeed, we are mirrors of our own most incredible love.

And since we dedicated this book to me AND you...

What if curiosity were *your* ticket, like it was mine?

What if dipping a toe into your *own* aliveness is what saves *you*?

THE TOOL

Okay, okay, I've been told I ask a lot of questions. That used to stop me dead in my tracks. Now? I accept the feedback and shift my approach. I don't dim my love for knowledge and the experience before me. I simply embody an alternative approach to finding answers, up to and including doing nothing.

Doing nothing?! Yes.

Silence. Rest. Pause. Marinate. STFU and listen. Discern.

Think out loud with me, ya?

In this same vein of easy-does-it noodling, what if your voice doesn't have to wait to come back in a lightning bolt? What if it could return in fragments? In shaky sentences? In whispers you're not sure are worth saying?

What if reclaiming your voice and being aligned in who *you* are isn't about being loud, but about being honest?

"Be authentic, even if your voice is shaking," isn't a slogan, my fellow brave human.

It's a practice. One that asks you to risk being real *before* you feel ready. One that reminds you: your voice doesn't get stronger by staying silent until it's perfect. It gets stronger by being used.

Here's what I'm learning to do:

- I speak before I'm fully polished.
- I pause when I catch myself performing for someone's approval.
- I tell the truth, even if I have to walk away to gain my composure, and even if my voice shakes upon my return.
- I trust that the people meant for me can handle my full volume—awkward pauses, broken sentences, shaky truths, guffaws, and all.

So now I'm asking you:

Can you say one *unrehearsed* thing today? This might look like:

- Saying no, even if your voice and hands shake.
- Recording a vulnerable voice memo to yourself, no filter... and then listening to it and being the person you need in that moment.
- Speaking of needs, try naming a need instead of swallowing it. Here's a lightweight script you can lift: "I'm feeling nervous, and this might not come out eloquently. I need to share something, though, do you have a few minutes?"

Let your voice be messy. Let your discoveries be clunky. Come out sideways if you need to!

Even upside-down is not failure. That's practice. That's remembering what it's like to be your true, unfiltered self.

You don't need a stage to reclaim your voice. You need a little courage and a lot of grace.

And most of all—*you need you*.

So, hey, now can you think out loud with me about what it would feel like to say the thing you've been holding in?

To not wait for the perfect time?

To speak like someone who finally believes in herself? Himself? Themself? Us?

Because your voice isn't something you earn, beautiful friend, it's yours to use in all its frequencies and symphonies with others.

And you don't have to get it right. You just have to speak.

Ya know, say it anyway.

I didn't for far too long. I thought no one was listening.

I guarantee you—someone is.

Hold up the mirror, and you'll see. You need to hear it as much as I do.

The You in every equation, after all, is also Me.

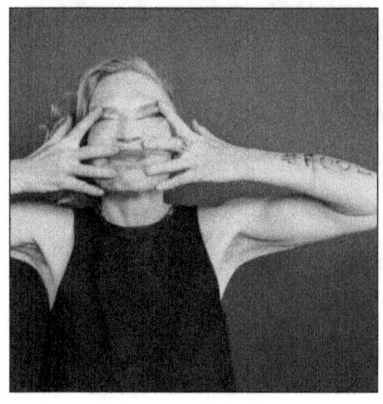

Amongst other adventures in engaging the world around her, **Natalie Petersen** hosts *Think Out Loud With Me*, a healthy dialogue with interesting humans that aims to ask questions most people dodge—easy ones with hard answers, and hard ones with no easy way out. It's messy meets a career-long media professional who knows how to hold a good conversation. Listen in and maybe, just maybe, get a little more honest with yourself.

Think Out Loud With Me streams live weekly and is available on all podcast directories. Join the conversation at https://1qr.com/tolwm.

CHAPTER 2

The Awareness Advantage

Discover and Heal Past Trauma

Susan Schiller

"Stay open. Don't close." I read these workshop notes, and I'm transported back to my yoga posture and my body's internal space.

Where are the tight places? Can I breathe and release further?

I close my eyes and feel my feet on the earth and my body as part of the ocean of consciousness, the unified field. Fully held, no fear.

I'm deeply grateful for this moment and the sense of lightness I feel. I reflect on the process of release that I've experienced repeatedly on my journey to healing from childhood trauma. My father violated my body, and as a result, I built protective layers that shielded me from feeling the trauma for more than eight years. However, these layers also silenced my voice and closed my heart. Decades have passed, and I can now affirm that healing unfolds in layers, and each released layer is progressively liberating.

Why is it difficult to open? Why is trauma often considered too painful to discuss? Our bodies hold these experiences for us, while our minds create narratives that allow us to construct a life in which trauma seems absent. However, our body doesn't forget; it stores the emotions for us.

Consider the innocence reflected in a child's eyes. They don't turn away in shame, as they haven't developed an internal dialogue to shut down reception of experience in the moment. That's where pure joy exists, and that is our birthright.

Take a deep breath and visualize a baby's innocence and joy. This story aims to guide us there.

MY STORY

I joined the Hare Krishna Movement in 1976 at age 16. I transitioned from a life under my father's control to one that required conformity and obedience to the temple rules. My new life emphasized chanting the Hare Krishna mantra, memorizing Vedic verses, and following strict vows—no meat, no illicit sex, no intoxication, and no gambling. It felt safe, and I could embrace this new life in the temple with a different persona. I believed studying the Vedic scriptures and sincerely chanting the Hare Krishna mantra would solve my problems in the material world.

I dedicated myself to temple life and service, becoming skilled in distributing books and fundraising for the temple. By 1981, I regarded myself as an advanced devotee. I agreed to an arranged marriage and continued my devotional service alongside my spouse.

Three years later, my husband and I traveled to meet my father with his new wife and their two sons for the first time. I felt confused and so disoriented after the visit. I hadn't seen my father for eight years and hadn't come to terms with him on my reasons for leaving. I felt unwilling to let him into my world and only said positive things about him to my husband. My father supported the movement, which was rare at the time.

THE CONVERSATION THAT CHANGED EVERYTHING

"Why do you feel stressed about this visit with your father? You've always spoken highly of him as a Krishna-conscious man," said my close devotee friend at the time.

What do I say? How do I explain my anxiety and distraction at having seen my father with his youngest son, my half-brother? The way he cozied up to him and the cute things he said reminded me of being his little daughter.

"Well, we just didn't have a good relationship," I muttered.

"What does *that* mean? You've always said he was a spiritual person. Isn't he proud of what you're doing now? Aren't you happy to see your new brothers? What's going on?" she pressed.

Panic came in waves, like milk boiling over—sudden, uncontrollable, and impossible to contain.

What will she think? Can I really say this?

But I had no one else. I had to let it out. Maybe she could help.

Looking down, I said quietly, almost ashamed, "He used to have sex with me."

I couldn't say more. The details were buried, repressed for so long they no longer had words.

To this day, she remembers the shift in me—how my whole presence changed as those seven words escaped my mouth. The weight of what I revealed hit her like a wave, just as it had crashed through me.

"You know, that was child abuse, and you should get help to deal with that," she said gently.

Child abuse? Those words hit me hard as I finally dropped into the pain I spent years avoiding.

I scheduled an appointment with a counselor. During these meetings, my repressed emotions surfaced, and my mind felt like a blur because I didn't feel secure enough to step outside the confines of the Hare Krishna way. I panicked and couldn't absorb what she was saying. After three sessions, I decided to cancel.

I'm not ready to talk about this.

Our son was born in 1984. The joy of being new parents is life-changing, and we felt it. The innocence of the child, those eyes full of wonder, created such a loving bond. We wanted the best for our family, so we moved out of the temple.

We started a bookkeeping business with a referral from one of the devotees. We got an apartment in another town. Other devotees lived nearby, but no temple structure or leaders dictated our daily schedule.

I no longer had any external structure to rely on. The instincts I developed to keep myself safe began to resurface. My attention was on everyone but myself; I was focused on ensuring my husband was happy and my son was well taken care of. I felt like a nervous wreck for a year and a half.

LEARNING TO LIVE

My body let go of everything—grief, fear, confusion—as I sobbed uncontrollably in the shower. Emotions poured out like a storm, and I could no longer hold back.

I feel lost. I don't know how to live.

Falling apart is messy. But our bodies carry an innate wisdom, a natural capacity to heal. We can trust that. When we allow emotions to move freely, we begin the process of releasing old patterns, making space for transformation, and a new way of living.

I began to feel the ground beneath my feet. In place of emotional turmoil, a quiet desire for self-worth began to take root.

I know I'm capable. I didn't finish high school because my father pulled me out. Now, I can make my own choice and do something about it.

I felt my confidence return, and I got my GED. I worked and took evening classes, resulting in an associate's degree in accounting and a bachelor's degree in computer science. I became a successful professional.

I delved into spiritual teachings like Deepak Chopra's *Seven Spiritual Laws of Success* and *Creating Affluence*. I practiced these teachings, and they worked (so I thought). Manifesting wealth in the external world felt great, but my body was still on edge. It was as if I had a dual persona; the professional side flourished while the personal side remained unaddressed.

Subtle resentment still reverberated through my body while making love. I fell into a pattern of submission rather than acting with intention. I didn't know how to honor myself in the relationship. How could I? *What does love really mean?*

My husband became the focal point of my anxiety. His problems became my problems. My safety was in making sure he was happy. Only later did I realize I constructed a prison for myself based on echoes of patterns from my relationship with my father.

HOW DOES HEALING UNFOLD?

When you open yourself to receiving answers, books, counselors, new friends, and life experiences often appear at just the right time. Your inner guidance system gives meaning to these encounters, allowing new awareness to arise from them. But for inner guidance to truly work, you must loosen your attachment to habitual thought patterns and begin retraining the mind.

Pay attention when a book that once inspired you begins offering fresh insights—those moments are signals from your inner radar. Also, notice when it's time to move on, when a new teaching or book calls you forward, signaling the need for a deeper layer of understanding. Trust this inner knowing, and don't be afraid to release what no longer supports your growth.

As I reflect on my own journey, I once believed I could go deeper using the mind alone. But thoughts alone cannot access the hidden spaces within the body. Practices like deep breathing, meditation, and resonant sound reach those places, helping to release stored trauma that lies beyond conscious awareness. The next part of this story is an example of that unfolding integration.

A PROFOUND MESSAGE FROM THE PAST

In 2017, my father passed away. Six years later, I took custody of his writings. I felt ready to explore my past without the emotional burden. A cassette recording of a conversation between my father and me from 1976 surfaced.

I eagerly played this time capsule for the first time, not knowing what to expect. Here are snippets:

Dad said, "What, are you recording again?"

My 15-year-old voice said, "Yeah, it'll be interesting to play back later."

I continued: "You know, I can see how childhood affects one's life. It shapes your whole consciousness. You know, it's like you're building a storehouse, a library, during that period with which to build your life. It's our foundation, like that story in the Bible about building the structures of houses. You know, if one is built on sand, it's bound to collapse; the water will come and wash it away. But the house built on a foundation of stone—solid truth—solid rightness stands forever."

Oh my God, I had such profound wisdom at that time. My voice was calming, inviting us to return to a state of peace even after a disturbing incident.

I said to Dad, "Life is a silly thing. One day things just seem so great, and the next day you have so much to learn, you just can't grok it. We've got to realize we're proceeding to the promised land, and we'll always have these things to work on. But the love we have is perfect. Perfect devotion to one another."

Hearing my voice after 45 years brought everything flooding back.

How was it possible that I still felt a perfect love for my dad? My mother had moved on with her life—without including me. Wasn't I the one left behind, trapped in it all?

I remember how I tried to stay on Dad's good side—the calm, thoughtful, philosophical side—because his other sides weren't safe.

AWARENESS RISING

During a restorative yoga retreat a year ago, I experienced a more physical integration of the memory.

We practiced heart-opening restorative yoga poses, deep breathing, and stretching. In the final relaxation pose, I felt a tight sensation in my chest that I wished would go away.

I know there's no medical reason for this sensation; one of those stored trauma layers is making itself known to me.

Tears rolled down my cheeks as I tried to let go.

Why won't this feeling disappear? I want it to go away!

The idea came: *It's time to give a voice to my younger self.* I thought about that recording from the archives that I hadn't shared with anyone except my husband.

Can I ask my close friends to listen to it?

I checked my phone and was excited to find the recording accessible without my computer. I arranged for my four friends to listen to it with me.

After explaining the context, we sat together and listened to the voice of the brave young girl I had once been. Their reactions said it all. Any mother would have wanted to protect her child—but mine had abandoned me. This time, though, I wasn't alone. I was surrounded by four women who stood with me—my advocates, my support.

I felt powerful in this special container with my advocates and freely expressed myself through a scream that allowed my inner child to emerge. She was finally heard after 45 years.

I felt a greater sense of freedom as we practiced qigong outside. Feeling the grass beneath my bare feet, I let out a yell as my arms circled and pressed forward, releasing through sound. I allowed Mother Earth to absorb my voice.

After this release, I still felt that tightness in my chest. The retreat leader advised me, "Instead of trying to eliminate trauma, see it as a crack in a boulder. Over time, moss and ferns take their places in the crack, reflecting nature's resilience. Embrace the crack, fill it with love, and let it blossom into wisdom."

The tension went away shortly after the retreat concluded.

After this experience, the phrase "Stay open, don't close" took on a deeper meaning. Healing doesn't come from resisting past trauma but from acknowledging it with an open heart. Let go of the narrative that keeps you trapped in a victim mindset. Stay open to new perspectives, ways of seeing your life story that offer freedom, not limitation.

But what about the perpetrator? There are always two sides to every story. Why would a father cross boundaries with his daughter, and how can such a thing be forgiven? In reading my father's autobiography, I discovered he, too, suffered childhood trauma. That insight opened my eyes to the generational impact of pain and to the truth that I'm here to break the cycle.

I invite you to consider that your life holds its own deep wisdom. This shift in mindset empowers you to move beyond victimhood. Trust your body's innate healing intelligence. Feel into your inner space and allow emotion to rise and release. This is not weakness, it's growth. This is the awareness advantage: when the mind quiets enough for the body to lead, true healing becomes possible.

FEELING MORE SPACIOUS

What is it like to live in the body without stored patterns and instinctual reactions?

There's simply more space, and the breath goes deeper. Colors appear vibrant, allowing one to notice the intricate beauty of nature like a child witnessing a flower for the first time. With the maturity and skills of an adult paired with the open heart of a child, life becomes rich. Stillness is within reach. You feel joy, and your access to gratitude is deep. Life energy flows through you with ease.

You can hear what your family member says without all the mind chatter. Mind chatter creates density, closing your perception of what is. (e.g., *How can he say that when he did that thing yesterday? Why didn't he consider my feelings?*) Accumulated layers of resentment or reflexive behaviors no longer occupy precious space.

You begin to take the lead in your own life, not bound by obligations to make others happy, to feel safe. You can access creativity and complete tasks with greater efficiency.

Your mind becomes your servant, not your defense mechanism.

This lightness is visible to others because you're open. Pure joy is accessible, and you just need to open to the journey.

THE TOOL

The practice outlined below will help you navigate your emotions through art and visualization. It provides a way to quiet your mind, allowing you to breathe deeply and open up your inner guidance. Gratitude is the key to fueling the positive changes that are on the horizon, as long as you choose to embark on this journey.

HEALING HAND PRACTICE

- Set an intention for your practice. Is there a situation or problem you would like to resolve? Write this down.
- Take a piece of paper or a page of your journal. Trace your hand. From the tracing, add fingernails, color, and any other artistic touches or decorations you like.

This is your healing hand. It will always listen to you. Let it represent your inner guidance that is always with you.

- On a journal page, write down the thoughts circling in your mind right now that cause you stress, anxiety, or unresolved feelings.
- Read back what you wrote and add anything you missed so the writing thoroughly represents what's circling in your mind.
- What emotion do you feel when you read the words back?
- Write down that internal dialog and capture that emotion.

Examples: cheated, angry, brokenhearted, anxiety, fear, stress, too much to do, lonely.

When you put your thoughts in writing, you have no need to hold them in your mind, thus allowing the mind to become still enough to proceed to the next part.

- Lie down flat or sit up with your back straight. Close your eyes and take deep breaths into your lower abdomen, exhaling slowly with the exhale—twice as long as the inhale.
- Notice the sensations in your body. Where do you feel tension or tightness?
- Place your healing hand on that area and apply gentle pressure. If unsure, you can rest your hand just above your heart.
- Breathe deeply and let out a sigh. Continue to breathe deeply, feeling your hand's warmth.
- As you do this, think about any memories that surface related to your current emotions.
- When you feel ready, open your eyes and write down your thoughts.

Notice any recurring pattern of thought in your internal dialogue. How can you release this pattern of judgment? How can you quiet your mental dialogue so you stay present and remain open?

- Visualize your ideal future. Remember, this change only requires you to focus on yourself.

- Breathe deeply. Write down your vision.

- Next, reflect on what you're grateful for right now. Recognize the abundance around you—air, water, and the simple things we often overlook.

- Write about what brings you joy. Let your gratitude flow.

Repeat this practice. Use your healing hand and ask your inner guidance for answers. Be open, and the personal connections and teachings you need will come.

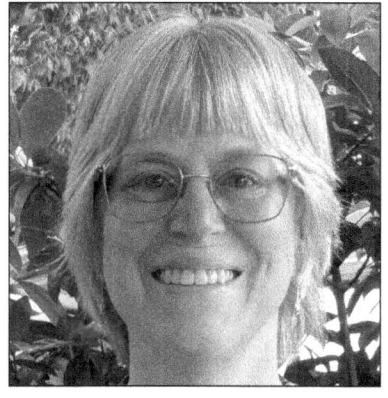

Susan Schiller is retired from the working world after a 35-year career. Her profession spanned accounting and accounting systems integration during the internet startup boom, financial systems project management for the government, and running a family-owned personal tax business.

Susan is the founder of Earth Rainbow Bridge, a nonprofit connection portal for healing inspiration. She's a mesa carrier and student of the Q'eros Nation's Pampamesayoq earth healing tradition in Peru.

She's dedicated to the art of meditation. She practices yoga, breathwork, and sound healing, and finds joy in sharing these practices.

Susan and her husband of 44 years live in Blowing Rock, North Carolina, and love hiking. They're both active in the community. She's an accomplished musician and plays piano and flute. She's also a creative weaver and knitter, making clothes for friends as an artful healing practice, weaving positive intentions with colorful yarn.

Connect with Susan:

Website: https://earthrainbowbridge.org

Email: sschiller2167@gmail.com

CHAPTER 3

I Am Not My Trauma

Moving Past the Victim and Reclaiming Your Divinity

Kim Louise Eden

Where there is ruin, there is hope for a treasure.

~ Rumi

MY STORY

I feel the tightness creeping up like a boa constrictor wrapping its cool body around me, slowly squeezing the breath from my lungs. My eyes slide over to the clock.

Yep, 4:58. It's almost time.

I hear the mechanical groan of the garage door reverberate through the house. A cold sweat pours over my body. My heart starts to race, pounding against my ribs like an insistent drumbeat. I try to sit still, pretending to be absorbed in the flicker of the television, but the thudding of my pulse drowns out all the sound.

Thud, thud, thud is all I can hear. My heartbeat hammers in my head. I feel like I'm going to explode, black out, and vomit all at once. I want to run, I want to hide, but I sit there and wait.

Thud, thud, thud.

"Momma?" My daughter's soft voice breaks through the cacophony inside my head. She bounds down the stairs.

"Can I go to my friend's house?"

"No, honey," I manage to say, my voice trembling with an edge of desperation. "You need to stay here."

With a heavy sigh, she mumbles, "I never get to go anywhere," as she turns and stomps away, her disappointment palpable. Little does she know that her presence anchors me, her small frame a lighthouse in a storm no child should ever have to witness. She's a fragile shield against the monster I married. He's still horrible when she's home, but the abuse is limited to verbal, versus more physical when she isn't home.

The door creaks open, and there he is, an unstable enigma. *Who will walk through tonight: the kind man I once knew, or the all-too-familiar tempest?* My husband, the boy I loved since childhood, the first boy I ever kissed, turned into a stranger capable of both tenderness and terror. Years of shared history can't mask the cracks that deepened into chasms. He's twisted and capable of dark deeds. Not only has he threatened me, but some of my beloved animal companions died under mysterious circumstances.

"Where's Anna?" he grumbles, dropping his rucksack with a careless thud.

"Upstairs," I reply, my voice barely audible over my racing thoughts.

Dinner is uneventful, an illusion of normalcy painted over the fractures in our lives. Yet, I know this isn't sustainable. He wasn't always abusive like this, but multiple tours overseas to active war zones warped him into a monster who slowly lost his grasp on reality. The therapist's warnings echo in my mind.

"Get out," she said. "He'll only get more dangerous if he knows you're leaving."

She was right. I knew it. The only thing that keeps me safe is knowing he won't risk his military career. I have no doubt he's capable of killing me. It wouldn't be fast; he would take his time to enjoy it.

While he works, I pack bags in secret, vacuum-packing and stashing essentials in hidden corners. Every item tucked away feels like a tiny stitch in the fabric of my escape plan. I tell everyone who needs to know: my boss, my daughter's daycare provider, and a friend in Tennessee who promised me sanctuary.

The day of departure arrives, a whirlwind of panic and adrenaline. I wait until after his lunch break before springing into action. I race through the house, grabbing bags, stuffing them into the car, and glancing over my shoulder as though his shadow might suddenly appear. My heart pounds relentlessly, a drumbeat of urgency and fear. I know that at any moment, he'll come home and discover my plan. The car is finally packed, and I'm off to get Anna and make our grand escape.

"Momma, why are the dogs in the car?" Anna asks, her curious gaze locking onto mine.

"We're going to visit friends in Tennessee," I say, forcing a smile. She doesn't question further.

As the miles stretch behind us, the suffocating grip of fear begins to loosen. The call comes late at night, his voice a mixture of fury and disbelief, but by then, I've already crossed into Tennessee, a step closer to safety, my friend's home a sanctuary after the storm.

Days turn into weeks, and amidst the haze of newfound freedom, I meet someone new. He's ready to be my shining knight, and I'm ready to be rescued.

Little do I know, I'm starting the cycle all over. One of my teachers frequently says, "We marry our wounds."

My new relationship lasts 12 long years. He's never physically abusive but is deep in addiction for most of our relationship, and I'm his codependent enabler.

I don't realize how much the narcissism and gaslighting eat away at the core of who I am. As an empath, I'm consistently silencing my inner knowing and believing his lies. This is the razor that splits me from my gifts and my identity. I realize that in my relationships, I give too much of myself. I've lost the core of who I am. People become my refuge and my addiction, leaving me hollow. This is my rock bottom.

There's nothing left of me; I'm a husk, a shell. How can I expect him to love me when there's nothing left to love? I have no clue who I am, what I like, or what I want in life.

It's time to turn inward, to face the demons I've danced with for years. Solitude becomes my medicine, and slowly, I begin to shed the layers of codependency and learn to love the fragments of myself I long ignored.

I dive deeper into plant medicine to help me on my healing journey. During one of my journeys, I go deep into the well of myself, and it's a gift. I sit with my darkness. I'm shown the parts of myself that long for love and attention—these pieces that chase the light of the day but are shamed and rejected, hidden from the world like dirty little secrets.

I was supposed to be all light and love, right?

Within myself is this rawness. I see demons, scary things, horrid faces, rotting flesh, the melting mask I use to face the world, and deep darkness. It's that thing that goes bump in the night, the thing behind you that makes you want to run before it touches you with its cold, dead hands, distorted by the ravages of time.

I have no fear; I'm curious, and that darkness responds in kind. I sit with it, befriending it, seeking to understand what it is and what it wants, and it simply wants love.

These are the deep, forgotten pieces of myself—the hated pieces. In my scramble to be enlightened, I forgot I must love this darkness in me.

A bird's song can't be one tone; we can't all be high-pitched. It needs its base tones to even out the high ones. I can't be light all day, all the time. In the darkness there's beauty, a resonance that adds to the beautiful song that is this world.

It's those pieces of me that need love, nurturing, and the understanding that yes, just as much as there's light within me, there is a darkness. As Carl Jung said, "The brighter the light, the darker the shadow."

I'm no longer ashamed of that darkness. It's a part of me that makes me beautiful. I realize that's what I've sought, pushed for, tried to find, but couldn't. That separation from this side of me is what blocked me from my divinity.

Duality is a song of highs and lows, and now I can see the dance. Once I embrace this part of my soul, I'm able to flow, to be as the wind and the breeze lifting the birds to new heights, the water in the calm pools finding its way to raging rivers and eventually to the ocean, recognizing that there are moments of chaos and order, seasons of warmth and cold, day and night. I am all those, and now I dance to the music, heart overflowing.

THE TOOL

"Your cracks can become the most beautiful part of you."

~ Candice Kumai

In Japan, there's an ancient art called kintsugi. It's a process of repairing broken pottery with gold. Kintsugi is a beautiful, artistic process, but it's also a powerful ceremony to grieve what was—and to find and celebrate the beauty and resiliency in the wound left behind. It's not about hiding the cracks, but displaying them in the glorious art of who you are in the dance of life.

To start this ceremony, bring to mind what you're currently healing, or what needs attention. Look for something you don't mind breaking that's tied to the event or person. If you don't have something at home, you can go to Goodwill or a similar thrift store and find something to represent the current struggle.

Once you have the piece, give gratitude for the process and envision pouring into it the different feelings you are experiencing.

Hold the object close to your heart and close your eyes. Focus on the event you are working through. Once you have a visual of the event or person, drop the item or hit it with a hammer so it breaks. Please be mindful to wear the proper protective equipment. As you collect the pieces, think about the different pieces of yourself that feel broken.

Once you have all the parts, it's time to wash them. As you wash them, observe the jagged edges, the big pieces, and the small pieces. Nurture these pieces and be gentle with them, as they can cut and hurt you unintentionally. Ask how these pieces represent who you are now.

This is a great opportunity to journal as everything dries. I like to set the broken pieces outside to warm in the sun.

Once everything is dry, you can start the process of reassembling the pieces. There are a few ways you can do this. You can buy a kit online with the glue, or you can use a thicker epoxy from an art supply store. I like to use epoxy and put in different colors of glitter. The traditional kintsugi method uses gold dust or gold leaf.

As you glue the pieces, call your energy back to you.

Example: *I call my energy back—the part of me that was hurt when you cheated. I love you and honor your hurt.*

This is a process of finding beauty in the hurt.

Once the process is done, you'll support some of the pieces as they heal (cure) with tape. Before I apply the tape, I write the different support structures I have on the tape. Example: *My community.*

At this point, give the piece time, recognizing it needs time to heal. Use it as a reminder that we, too, need to give ourselves grace and time to heal.

Once your kintsugi piece is completed, give gratitude to the piece for the journey you started together. Display it proudly.

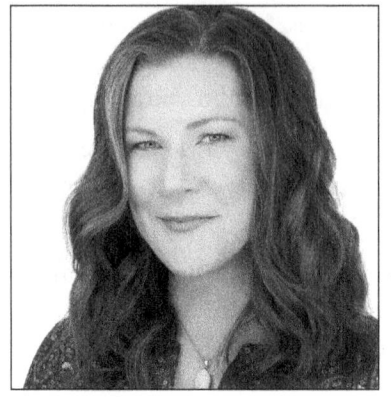

Kim Eden is an intuitive empath, PSYCH-K® Practitioner, Reiki Master, NLP practitioner, holistic herbalist, hypnosis practitioner, life coach, and ordained minister. These are just labels. The reality is, she's an energetic being having a human experience, and simply *is*. She feels it's her purpose in life to be the vessel that light shines through. To offer hope to the hopeless.

Kim grew up on a rural desert farm in southern Arizona. She spent most of her childhood lost in her imagination. The open desert was her playground; her best friends were her horses, dogs, goats, and cats that called the farm home.

Growing up, Kim was always the oddball and outcast. She saw the world differently, even at a young age. She could see the energy that flowed into everything. She realized she was called to help and could hold that space for others.

Kim doesn't believe one modality will heal everything. This belief has led her to learn different modalities. For over 25 years, she has worked on her spiritual development. She has attended courses at Arthur Findlay College to study mediumship and psychic development, and has numerous certifications and additional training in holistic modalities, energy psychology, and energy work. She has traveled to learn with shamans, maestros, and healers throughout North and South America.

Kim credits Stephanie Urbina Jones and Jeremy Pajer at Freedom Folk and Soul for giving her a solid foundation. She's grateful to Miguel Kavlin at Sacha Runa in Bolivia for his retreat, which allowed her the space for healing.

Connect with Kim:

Email: keden.peacefulpath@gmail.com

Facebook: https://www.facebook.com/peacefulpathinnerillumination

YouTube: https://www.youtube.com/@peacefulpath1866

CHAPTER 4

Vibrations of Calm

Using Breath and Sound to Reset Your Nervous System

Sharon Cassidy, PT, DPT, MPH

MY STORY

Oh God, what the hell.

I found an empty bathroom in the hallway outside the ICU and just made it to the toilet before I threw up.

That was close.

When I opened the door to leave, my friend, Hunter, one of the orderlies, was standing in the hallway looking at me.

"You alright?" he asked, looking skeptical.

"Yeah, I just had an upset stomach. I'm good," I answered.

On my break, I went across the street to the cafe for a cup of coffee and sat at the counter. Hunter came in and sat next to me. He leaned in close and looked me in the eye.

"Are you pregnant?"

"No. Why would you say that?" I said, alarmed.

Hunter went on. "Because that's not the first time you threw up today, and you've been looking queasy. I've got three kids, so I know the signs."

"No, I don't have any reason to be pregnant. So no," I said, leaning away from him.

I gave my doctor a urine specimen for a pregnancy test yesterday. The results would take a day or two.

I was a single 20-year-old college student, working as a nurse's aide in the intensive care unit at a hospital in New Orleans. My mother was the head nurse. She wasn't working that day, so I didn't expect to see her.

"Sharon, Dr. Goldman said he has your test results. He wants you to come to his office this afternoon when you get through here," the nurse informed me.

"Okay," I said as my stomach dropped and my heart raced.

When I got to his office, I sat in the waiting room.

"He'll see you in his office in just a minute," the nurse said.

"Okay," I answered.

God, why is it so cold in here? He's going to tell me, and that's it. One word—yes or no—and then everything changes.

What if it's yes? What then?

My heart pounded, but I tried to be calm.

This could be a life sentence. Jesus. Please be no. Just no.

"You can go in now," the nurse said.

Breathe, just breathe.

My legs shook, and my hands grew slick with sweat.

Here goes.

I opened his office door.

"Mom?!" I exclaimed.

All the blood drained from my face, and it felt like ice rushed to my feet. She looked shocked and sad, her hands folded in her lap.

Neither of us spoke. *What can I say? What does she want to say?*

The room was thick with tension.

My mind raced.

Dr. Goldman sat behind his desk and said, "You're about six weeks."

Why did he ambush me like this? I'm not a child. I should be the one to tell my parents.

In 1969, abortion was illegal in New Orleans. It was also illegal for single women to be prescribed birth control pills. My mother was friends with Dr. Goldman. They worked together at the hospital.

"Can you help?" she asked, looking at Dr Goldman with hope.

I held my breath.

He hesitated, looked at his hands resting on his desk, and then, with resignation, "No," he said.

That was that.

We went home. I went to my room. I stood in front of my dresser mirror only to see someone I didn't recognize.

Will I have to go into a "home"? Will I have to drop out of school and quit my job? Hide? Be sent away?

I wasn't ready to be someone's mother. I wasn't ready to carry the shame and guilt, the anger and grief. I didn't want my life dictated by a mistake. And no, having a baby and giving it up for adoption wasn't an option I wanted to consider. I wanted no part of the overt, insidious judgment woven into the fabric of my Catholic-dominated culture.

My mother was in shock, and so was I. She called my father at work and told him I would pick him up. I felt out of body, trying to maintain a normal composure. I don't think he suspected the seismic shift that would happen when we got home.

Mom waited for us in the formal living room. "Come sit," she said.

By now, Dad must have expected something severe. We never used the formal living room.

"Sherry's pregnant," she said.

Once again, the air in the room pressed in on me like a heavy weight. I barely breathed, waiting for someone to say something to break the oppressive tension I felt.

"I still love you," my dad said, looking at me with kindness.

My classmate, the father, brought information about an abortion clinic in Puerto Rico. My mother went with me.

It was done. I came home, and we never talked about it.

I went to school, had a life, pushed through, pushed past.

Or so I thought.

I didn't realize it then, but my body held the unsaid, the unseen, the unloved parts of that story. Part of me stayed frozen. I buried my feelings and silenced my guilt, shame, and anger.

But these feelings don't stay buried. And while I learned to function, to achieve, even to help others heal, I had yet to turn inward and truly listen.

It would take years, layers of physical symptoms, and the steady crumbling of all the ways I kept myself armored before I realized healing could only happen when I listened and surrendered to the messages my body kept trying to give me—messages that allowed me to find my way to a balance.

And that's what brought me here.

To the jungle.

THE DIALOGUE

I just knew I had to come to the jungle. There was something I could only get by being here. But I don't know yet what it is.

Something has changed in me lately. I feel open, receptive, calm. I'm surprised by my peace.

There you are, my body whispers.

At 5:15 a.m., the jungle erupts in spectacular voice.

"Waaaaaaaaaaaa!" It goes on for minutes at a deafening pitch.

I don't know who started it, but every bird, reptile, mammal, and insect joins in with gusto, creating a raucous symphony that makes me laugh out loud and shout with joy.

It's a great big, "Hallelujah, I claim this day!"

I spend hours pummeled by waterfalls, soaking in the quiet pools of roaring rivers, and lying prone on giant, sun-warmed boulders. The voices of the falls and the river fill me with an exquisite calm. I feel completely awake, present, home.

As my body surrenders to the boulder's mass, I press my forehead onto its warmth and hear its deep bass voice:

"Daughter, I'm glad you're here. Give me what burdens you. That is why I'm here. I will give it to the crystal waters to carry away."

I feel completely undefended. Safe. Whole.

I'm compelled to go to the river, get into the water, be pummeled and blessed, cleansed by the waterfall, and thrilled by its effervescence.

What if I show up with this marvelous gift of coalesced molecules and energy I call my "body," ready to experience life?!

Let me find the balance of *do* and *be*, the masculine and feminine in their highest forms.

It's been a long journey to this place. Like getting to the river, there's no path, but there is a way. It isn't easy to see how to proceed. Sometimes, I'm sure it's not possible. But I go anyway.

Between the roar of the river and the silence of surrender, I remember the companion I neglected, misunderstood, and too often silenced: my body.

She carried the weight of it all—the joy, the grief, the yeses I meant to say, and the no's I never could.

And now, she's ready to speak. I'm finally ready to listen.

That's when the dialogue begins.

You're different now, my body says with a hint of surprise.

I smile. "How so?"

You're softer, present. You're here with me. Not fixing, not pushing through, just feeling.

I let that sink in.

"You've been waiting a long time for this, haven't you?" I ask.

My whole life, she says softly. And then, *do you recall that time you were buried alive?*

"Vividly. Why?" I tilt my head curiously.

Because that was a version of how I've felt our whole life, until you could finally hear me and begin to understand what I've been trying to tell you.

"Go on," I say, taking a deep breath and letting it out slowly, remembering.

I'm wrapped in a shroud. It's tight. I can't move. I'm trying to be brave, but my heart's pounding. I'm gasping. Don't cover my face! They do, though. I start to panic.

They carry me to the gravesite. Don't bury me deep! Please. Not deep!

They put a breathing tube in my mouth and begin to cover me with sand. It's cold, heavy. My breath is ragged while they pile it on. I wiggle a little as the sand builds up. Three feet deep. I can't move. I'm rigid with tension.

I take several deep, hungry breaths.

And then, I just let go.

The distinction between who is speaking—my mind or my body—is only slight now.

I let my breath soften, slow, and smooth. Each inhale reaches deeper, brushing the edges of my fear, and each exhale carries it away like dust in the wind.

I begin to hum, low and steady. The sound vibrates in my chest at first, then spreads into my throat, down my spine, into the bowl of my pelvis. My bones start to hum back. It's as if I've struck a tuning fork at the center of my being.

The vibration moves like a wave through my muscles and fascia. My shoulders melt, and my belly softens. Thought recedes, replaced by tone.

I'm no longer just breathing.

I am the breath.

I am the sound.

In this resonance, my body is the tuning fork, tuned back to some remembered pitch of calm. In the presence of this vibration, I feel a wholeness—a cellular exhale, as if every cell is singing, *You are safe. You are here.*

That experience stays with me, a recognition that my body was always speaking.

And now, all these years later, I'm finally listening. This moment of surrender is a turning point.

I didn't fully understand it at the time, but my body's first clear message was:

I am with you. I have always been with you. But you have to hear me.

So, I listen—not just to symptoms or pain, but to the language beneath them. And as I do, the story of my fibroids rises to the surface not just as a medical diagnosis, but as a message my body tried to deliver for years.

This is where our real dialogue begins.

My body exhales deeply, then whispers, *You've unearthed the memory, but there's more to release. Do you remember when we carried the fibroids?*

"Yes. I do. But I didn't understand your message," I answered. "I thought finding them and removing them was the answer."

They weren't just physical, my body continues. *They were everything you buried inside. The things you swallowed. The truths you denied. The wild power you dimmed so you could survive.*

"You were trying to tell me I had a womb full of 'no's' that were never heard. They were my body's protest of unvoiced emotions, unmet needs, and the absence of joy," I realize out loud.

You called them tumors, she says quietly, *I called them messages.*

"I didn't receive the messages, even after they were removed twice. The third time, I had a hysterectomy. That was tough."

Yes, she says, hearing my thoughts. *And the surgeon took your ovaries too, without ever discussing it with you. She did that on her own. Grief and rage from that violation still have consequences for me.*

I pause, then go on.

"Yeah, I was castrated and gutted. I felt betrayed," I say out loud, touching the thick scar on my belly. "I just kept getting through it and moving on, but I wasn't moving on. Not really."

"I felt outraged at how I was disregarded. No one acknowledged the importance of this loss. It's not just my organs that were taken," I realize out loud.

"It was my identity as a woman and membership in a community of women.

"I grieved the loss of being whole."

You can't surgically remove the message by removing the tissue. That's why I kept growing the fibroids back, my body agrees matter-of-factly.

This experience pushed me to look deeper into healing. I felt hollowed out. I needed to find my way to the river. I needed to reclaim my sovereignty physically, emotionally, and energetically.

My body stretches and yawns.

Come with me. I want to show you something. We're going on a journey.

"Is there pain involved? Sandy graves?" I ask hesitantly.

Just come. You'll see.

THE JOURNEY

I'm seated in front of a shaman. She has an array of sound instruments in front of her. Between us is an altar. My body is relaxed and alert.

"Place your hands gently on your belly," she says. "Take a deep breath and hold it as long as you can. Now, exhale long and slow. Feel the space of your womb. It is still there energetically. Take another deep breath and hum into your womb space."

I continue to hum into my womb and breathe into the grief and pain that's still there, after all these years, wanting to be witnessed. I feel a liquid heat in my abdomen that rises through me like a cleansing flow.

My tears release grief, guilt, anger, and shame, and my healing begins.

It isn't immediate. But each breath is an offering. Each tone is a vibration of calm.

I sing into my womb like a cave, letting the sound bounce and echo. I let my breath expand and soften me from the inside out. With every exhale, every tone, the old weight of loss lifts.

The shaman helps me lie down, and the journey continues.

I feel safe and undefended. The feminine and masculine dance. They're like music weaving, spiraling, rising, separating, but never far apart.

Treble and bass.

Their energies are equally powerful with the feminine—huge, warm, soft, flowing. An irresistible force that can take any shape, go anywhere like water, like wind. The masculine is warmer and more concentrated, like fire and earth. Its power supports the feminine with deep bass tones that create an energetic structure in which the feminine draws into itself every particle, every element.

In this fertile space, everything is created and born into multiple dimensions. The masculine supports the feminine in a rich, sensual, integrated process of inclusion and abundance.

I'm in an alchemical process of converting the lead of indoctrination by culture, religion, and ancestry into the gold of my liberated, juicy, fully present self. I experience everything sung into existence. Every song contributes to a unifying chorale that creates our experience.

After the journey, I listen to the Dalai Lama chant. His tones and words create a fluid structure that draws me into sacred community.

All is possible.

THE TOOL

INTRODUCTION

Welcome to a dialogue with your body using your breath and voice. Your body is always speaking; this is a space to slow down, breathe deeply, and listen. Let this be a doorway to the rich world of breath and sound practices.

SECTION 1: PREPARING THE SPACE

Before you begin:

- Find a quiet, comfortable place where you can sit or lie down undisturbed.
- Take a few moments to arrive—feel your body supported by the earth.
- Place one hand on your heart, one on your belly. Close your eyes.
- Breathe gently. Let your awareness settle inward.

SECTION 2: BREATH AWARENESS PRACTICE

Practice: Breath Process

1. Inhale into the belly.
2. Expand into the ribs.
3. Lift into the chest.
4. Hold for as long as it is comfortable.
5. Now fully exhale a long, slow breath through your mouth.
6. And when you are fully exhaled, hold for as long as this is comfortable.
7. Repeat at least 5-7 times.

Reflection Questions:

- Where do I feel my breath moving most freely?
- Where does it feel restricted or tight?
- What does this tell me about how I'm holding or protecting myself?

SECTION 3: HUMMING PRACTICE

Practice: Grounding with Humming

1. Inhale deeply through the nose.
2. On the exhale, softly hum ("mmmm") with lips closed.
3. Play with varying tones and volume.

4. Feel the vibration in your face, throat, and chest.

5. Repeat for 3–5 minutes.

Reflection Questions:

- Where do I feel the vibration most clearly?
- Is there any place that feels numb or silent?
- What does my body want me to know about this area?

Body Dialogue Prompt:

"Dear [body part], I feel you vibrating (or not) here. What are you holding? What would you like to share with me?"

SECTION 4: VOICE TONING

Practice: Toning Vowels to Open Energy Centers

With your mouth open:

Choose a tone for each vowel and let it resonate in your body.

- AH (heart/chest)
- EH (throat)
- EE (eyes/head)
- OH (belly)
- OO (pelvis/legs)

Let your voice rise and fall naturally, with no pressure to sound "good." Play with toning different sounds; vary the volume. You can't do this wrong. Remember to prolong the sound on the exhale.

Reflection Questions:

- Which tones felt easiest or most natural?
- Which tones felt strained or hard to sustain?
- Did any emotions or memories arise?
- What is your body expressing through each sound?

SECTION 5: INTEGRATION AND JOURNALING

Closing Practice: Breath and Silence

Return to simple breath awareness. No sound now. Just listening.

Journal Prompts:

- What did I discover about how my body holds emotion or memory?
- Did any particular sound or tone bring relief, sadness, or joy?
- What message did I hear from within today?

Integration Practice:

Create a two-minute daily ritual:

- Three breaths, one minute of humming, one vowel tone.
- Close with a hand on your heart and ask: "What do you need from me today?"

I offer you this simple yet powerful tool in hopes that you'll step into your curiosity about your body's wisdom, creating a safe space to experience balance, harmony, and healing.

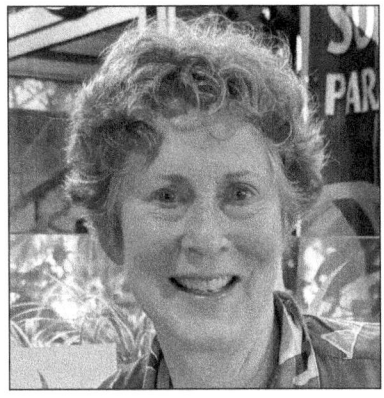

Sharon Cassidy has spent much of her life exploring how we heal—physically, emotionally, and energetically. Her journey began with traditional training in physical therapy, but it was craniosacral therapy that introduced her to the body's deeper intelligence. This path eventually led her to study with Peruvian shamans, who helped her understand that illness is often the body's way of speaking when we haven't listened.

In her own life, that conversation showed up as fibroids, thyroid issues, kidney disease, and skin cancer. For years, she tried to "fix" these issues through traditional medicine. True healing began when she slowed down and started listening.

Today, Sharon finds balance through Holotropic and Pranayama breathwork, as well as vocal practices like humming, toning, and chanting. These methods soothe the nervous system, helping to integrate physical and emotional experiences that otherwise trigger fight-or-flight responses and disconnect us from our bodies.

Through breath and sound, Sharon embodies and teaches a return to stillness and wholeness. She offers a grounded space to explore these practices—tools that can help you hear your body's messages and support your unique healing journey.

Sharon holds a Doctorate in Physical Therapy and a Master of Public Health from UNC Chapel Hill, and she has worked in healthcare for over 40 years. Her most profound lessons, though, came from learning to be present with herself.

She currently co-houses with two dear friends, Vicki and Rick, on thirteen acres in the North Carolina mountains, along with Sunny Love Dawg and her cats, Fergus and Queenie.

Connect with Sharon:

Email: scassidy144@gmail.com

Member of the Board of Directors of the Earth Rainbow Bridge organization: earthrainbowbridge.org

Mesa Carrier of Pachacuti and Pakarina Wisdom traditions

CHAPTER 5

The Emotion Map

Find and Inspire Joy Without Toxic Positivity

Amanda Fuel, Adoptive Mom and Public Speaker

MY STORY

I knew what to do; I just wasn't doing it.

And I needed to do it—right now—or lose my apartment, my freedom, and the business I worked so hard for.

I had quit my job six months ago and had been flying solo in my own business, teaching small group classes about stage presence. I even had a system that was working pretty well so far: I gave a talk, then followed up individually with interested parties. Not rocket science. Simple. Easy.

Or so it seemed.

So why was I still sitting here, stuck to the couch, watching *Grey's Anatomy* until even Netflix was getting concerned, asking me far too often, "Are you still watching this?"

I knew *exactly* how much *Grey's Anatomy* I watched this week alone, because I was housesitting for a mentor of mine. She was several steps ahead of me on this entrepreneurial path, so this week, I was literally surrounded by evidence that it was possible to make a good living teaching what I loved—and even own a home and travel the world.

One might think I would be extra-inspired living under her beautiful, high ceilings; relaxing against the luscious, matching burgundy pillows on her new, creamy white couches; or soaking in the giant, gleaming bathtub in the even giant-er master bath.

But that stark white "season three" lettering on the black screen in front of me told a different story. It showed that I'd sat here for nearly four seasons of this show, in this one week alone. And the worst part? I wasn't even enjoying it.

Binge-watching can be a delightful way to spend some downtime, but this was just the opposite—because I knew that, day by day, my funds were running out fast. Even after the payment for this housesitting gig, the numbers were clear: I had to sell several more spots in my new class to meet my bills this month.

But I was stuck—real good and stuck—and slowly becoming a new multi-colored pillow on that heavenly couch.

My eyes were also stuck, glued to Meredith Grey's eternally confused pout—except, why did my attention keep darting over to the bookshelf beside the TV? I brushed it aside.

I've read all those books already. That's why she's my mentor, because we love the same books.

But one of the books kept repeatedly grabbing my gaze and yanking my attention off the show. It was called *Ask and It Is Given*, a channeled work by Esther Hicks. First of all, the name itself was already challenging me. *Ask and it is given? I'm sure that's meant to be inspiring, but at the moment, that's just mean.* How could anyone have the nerve to believe you could just "ask" and it would simply be "given," let alone make it the title?

Eventually, and with a dramatic, nearly audible eye roll, I unglued myself from the couch and shuffled over in my slippers to pick it up. I'd read this book some months ago, so I started reluctantly flipping through the pages. That's when I found the list.

On page 114, there's a list of 22 emotional states, ranging from *powerlessness* to *joy/freedom*. On first glance, it's nothing new, just another list of emotions, but what struck me about it that day was one word at the top of the page:

THE EMOTION MAP • 47

Guidance.

It is called the Emotional *Guidance* Scale.

Huh. So maybe it's not just a list, I realized. I'd seen many lists like this, and they were great to help me name a feeling or two. But what I needed, in the middle of my *Grey's Anatomy* pity party, was indeed *guidance*!

I stared at the page—just a black and white list of 22 feelings that I felt completely lost in. But if this page was indeed offering me guidance, did that mean:

I can figure out where I currently am, and then **move***?*

And if so:

Is this a **map***?!*

The thought struck me powerfully as I sat back down with the book, feeling the page glowing and almost pulsing in my hands. *Where am I right now?*

I started looking way down at the bottom, because that's how I felt: stuck in a hole. But to my surprise, I found myself relating to words closer to the middle of the list. Words like *frustration* and *overwhelm* seemed to fit better.

Huh, I'm not as far down as I thought. Interesting. I felt one of my eyebrows lift, and a little spark of energy light up inside me.

Okay, so I guess I'm just stuck in frustration this week, hitting my head against a wall, steaming and stewing about it. So now what?

Frustration was number ten out of 22, so according to the list, it appeared I was very close to both *overwhelm*—below me at number 11— or *pessimism*, up at number nine. So *pessimism* was slightly *above* where I was. *Wait, what?!*

Pessimism? That awful word is actually above me on the scale? How can that be?!

I was thoroughly trained to *never* give in to pessimism—that there was always a bright side, always a "glass is 1/78th full" angle to be found. *How can pessimism be this far up on the list?*

But somehow, looking around the site of my week-long pity party, I realized the eternally optimistic part of me was certainly not in control right now. The frustrated part of me definitely had the wheel here. If I were going to move—literally *move* from this couch—this part needed to shift.

Could it be that it needed to move *toward* pessimism?

If I treated this list like a map, and if I wanted to move toward joy, then the path led right through pessimism. Annoying as that was, I decided to give it a try. I stared at the word, noticing how even just looking at it long enough was making me squirm, my mouth scrunching into strange shapes as I pondered it. What the heck was the feeling of pessimism?

I tried some phrases that I thought would match it:

"Nothing is going to get better."

"This is as good as it gets."

"Nothing I do will make a difference."

Yeesh. That all sounded so heavy.

*But what if this **is** as good as it will ever get? No, really, what if?*

I could feel that I was allowing myself to genuinely believe these thoughts!

My stomach turned.

But, to my surprise, my next thought didn't feel so bad: *If this is as good as it gets… is this truly all that bad?*

Sure, you're struggling to fill your classes and make ends meet, but maybe it's okay to struggle to build something great. Maybe all the confusion and rejection are just how it is right now, and it's not meant to be different at the moment.

Whoa! I felt my eyes open just a little wider, and something relaxed inside me. *Did I just move from frustration to pessimism **with my thoughts?** And wow, this pessimism place is more welcoming than I thought.*

It was as if I stumbled into a neighboring town everyone said was a run-down cesspool of thieving barbarians, but apparently, it was, well, a bit of a hidden gem. Admittedly, it was a tad gloomy, but with definite notes of *acceptance* and even some *relief* in the air. At the very least, it was a break from *frustration*.

I looked back down at the page, clutching to it like a tiny life raft. Above *pessimism* were some additional ominous words: *boredom* and then *contentment*. I was equally unfamiliar with those, but was it possible they held some hidden treasures in their folds as well?

As I worked with my new "map" that day, I began to feel my physical energy shifting, too. I was no longer glued to the couch. I found myself opening my laptop, engaging with my work, texting a few friends, and potential clients.

Occasionally, my attention drifted back down to phrases like, *"There's too much to do. I'm never gonna find enough people who can pay soon enough to make my rent."* But something was decidedly different this time.

I knew where that thought lived. It lived smack dab in the middle of *Overwhelm Town*, and if I could recognize it, it was as if I was finding the "you are here" point on the map—and that meant I could face the direction I wanted to travel and make it to any other point I wanted to go! Slowly but surely, I could get there.

When I noticed frustration or overwhelm had hold of the wheel, I didn't try to jump up into hope or passion. Rather, I slowly walked those parts of me through *pessimism* and *boredom* first, until I felt the gentle breeze of *contentment* whispering through my hair. Then, I knew the rest would easily flow.

Within just a couple of weeks, my class filled up. I got the venue settled, supplies paid for, and I even paid my rent on time. A miracle truly occurred!

In fact, multiple miracles occurred, and as I began using the map more frequently, I ended up adding many supplemental emotions to it. Finally, I created a horizontal graphic of it to remind me that this is not a hierarchy, and every emotion is just a new town along the roadway.

Dealing with the emotional ups and downs of an entrepreneurial journey was priceless to me at that time. It allowed me to stay in business for myself, teaching whatever I wanted to share, and speaking across the country, even as a highly sensitive, emotional person. However, it turned out I would need even greater emotional agility for what lay ahead: motherhood.

BECOMING AN ADOPTIVE MOM

In 2018, my husband and I welcomed a ten-year-old foster kiddo into our home. At the time, they were called Jewell and went by she/her pronouns. I felt an immediate soul-level connection to her, with her wild, untamed hair and crystal blue eyes, and we knew she would complete our family. However, we weren't prepared for the wide range of intense reactions and outbursts she would have, due to ten years of traumatizing situations.

One state that came up consistently for her was the feeling of *blame*. This was difficult for me to relate to; I was scolded away from blaming anyone else and taught to always take responsibility for my circumstances.

But Jewell taught me differently. When I considered *blame* as an emotional state rather than an action, I realized that it was surprisingly *higher up* on the map than *powerlessness* or even *anger*. So, Jewell wasn't completely giving up her power whenever she felt *blame*. Often, she regained it by reminding herself *she* wasn't inherently bad, and she still had inherent value and worth. Although this came from her early years, it surfaced repeatedly at our house.

One day, she walked in the door with her dad and immediately spilled a full, large, bright fuchsia smoothie all over our fresh white carpet. I reacted with knee-jerk high volume, which I tried hard not to use because it could quickly trigger her PTSD.

"Jewell! What happened?!"

With tears in her eyes, she yelled back, "It's not my fault! That wall attacked me!"

I stopped in my tracks. All I could hear her saying was, "I'm still good inside!" She was actually *mustering* strength, shaking off shame, and reminding herself she wasn't the (only) cause of pain. *Blame* was a tool, a direction where her inner anger could go to be released! It wasn't an emotion I needed to train out of her or try to stifle.

Rather, we soon recruited Craig-the-imaginary-roommate to take all the blame for minor mistakes and oversights throughout the home. "Craig forgot to put the silverware away again, Mom!" she would say. Or I would comment how cheeky Craig was for distributing Jewell's dirty socks all over the house. It was a way to playfully use her strong blame muscle for good, rather than trying to silence it.

If I hadn't been familiar with the gold from each emotional state, I'm not sure I could have built the trust we needed to become family, having met each other so much later in life. But I knew if I could name the emotion—sometimes only to myself—then she wasn't lost. I could always find her on the map, help her give voice to where she was, and occasionally lead her in the positive direction.

Between using this map for myself, my clients, and now my kiddo, I discovered a strange phenomenon. I was no longer afraid of my or others' emotions. Wherever they are on the scale, I can now locate them. I don't even need them to move up the scale or work their way to a different town. And my lack of resistance to every emotion helps them all feel welcome, and keeps us all out of toxic positivity without getting lost.

Today, I'm so proud of the strong bond my kiddo and I have forged that allows us to navigate choppy waters and outright hurricanes— everything from COVID homeschooling and international travel to my husband's traumatic brain injury.

While I've never thought of this as a tool to heal deep trauma, I consider it essential for dancing with the whole range of emotions that come with a full and fast-paced life. I use it regularly to help me show up as the mom, the speaker, and the human I want to be, without needing anyone to be in a different place than where they are right now.

Many thanks to *Grey's Anatomy* for keeping my eyes trained toward that bookshelf all those years ago!

THE TOOL

Link to the map: http://bit.ly/4kQ9I4z

The Map:

1. You Are Here: Locate Yourself on the Map
   a. What emotion do you feel when you think about something you deeply desire?

b. The larger "town names" may get you in the ballpark, but zoom in on the smaller "street names" within the towns to find the one that really hits home.

c. Go ahead and feel that feeling thoroughly. Let it out; you are not lost, you are here!

2. Become A Tourist: Find the Gifts of This Town

a. Every emotional state has a purpose to share, a gift to impart. Have a look around and find those "best-kept secrets" that feel meant just for you. You can see some of the gifts I've discovered below.

b. Remember, no matter how successful, rich, hot, famous, smart, or perfect you will someday become, you will *always* find yourself moving both up and down the map. This is the full range of human emotion, and no change of circumstance will save you from feeling *any* of it. So, let's get exploring!

c. Try to remove that extra layer of judgment about how you "should" or "shouldn't" feel and just accept that all these towns exist inside us all. Notice how encountering them on their own is a lot easier than visiting them with a heavy backpack of shame or pride.

- Gift of unworthiness and jealousy: something. At least I am pointed toward *something* I see as "good." I'm out of the dark corner of powerlessness. I am "unworthy" of _____, or I'm jealous of _____. I can at least see that someone, somewhere, has something kinda good. My desire flickers to life.

- Gift of revenge: focus/thinking. Okay, so I'm not willing to go off in a blind rage, unhinged. I want my energy to go toward something specific! My prefrontal cortex must turn on to determine the most satisfying way to get justice. How will I pull it off? If I have endless energy and nothing is off the table—thank you, rage— what will I focus on?

- Gift of disappointment: I tried. If I'm disappointed, that means I risked something—went after my desire—

and it didn't go my way. I dared to want, to dream, to act, to try. Now I know a few things that don't work to get it. If I can stomach this feeling for a minute, let it slow me down and teach me, I may just be able to try again.

3. Intentional Travel: Move One to Two Towns Toward Joy

   a. When ready, start to study the words of the neighboring town. It may not be one you've visited often, as we usually get stuck due to not being trained or allowed to feel all of these, like I did with frustration. Just gently lean toward it, rather than forcing it.

   b. Create some phrases that match that neighboring town and see if any ring a little bit true for you. Use your attention and focus to see if the stuck part of you will shift into genuinely believing the new thoughts or phrases.

   c. Listen for the gold within this new town. What does it hold for you? Do you feel a little relief just from getting out of the town that had you stuck? Are you willing to feel into this new town, just for a few moments?

4. Become Familiar and Fluent: Never Be Afraid of an Emotion Again

   • Play the Name Game and attempt to name your and others' emotions when they come up, letting them know you're okay with wherever they're at.

   • Visit the towns you're least familiar with intentionally, spending just one more minute in them than you usually allow yourself. Soon enough, you won't get stuck on your travels.

   • Reduce any need for toxic positivity as you lose your fear of any emotion and fully learn your way around.

While my love for world travel is strong, becoming familiar with my *inner* landscape has offered me the most freedom of all. May this map help you, inspire you, and free you, too!

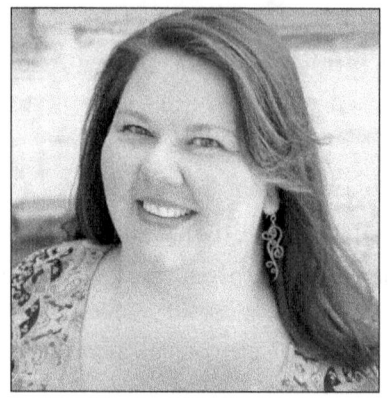

Amanda Fuel is the founder of Next Level Fuel, which develops innovative projects in the field of human empowerment. Amanda is an interactive speaker on a mission to disrupt the old norms of public speaking to include more uncommon voices and raw, authentic expression. She's also the mother of one wild child and three even wilder dogs, living in Northern Colorado where she enjoys biking, swimming, and hosting game nights or story shares.

You won't find Amanda in a kitchen if she can help it, but you can often find her doing art projects with a friend or continuing to teach her favorite class: Stage Presence for Thought Leaders.

Connect with Amanda:

Website: https://AmandaFuel.com

Facebook: https://www.facebook.com/amandafewell11

LinkedIn: https://www.linkedin.com/in/amandafuel/

CHAPTER 6

The Center that Holds

The Quiet Power of a Self-Remembered

Laurie S. Cossar

I am the still point and the spiral. I am the vessel and the light. I am the one I have been waiting to return to.

MY STORY

What are you prepared to do for your freedom?

The room was dim, heavy with the scent of unfamiliar linens and the silence that follows a storm. I sat on the edge of the hotel bed—knees drawn up, hands trembling—when my dear friend Sam knocked softly and let himself in. He had a way of entering without disrupting, like he already knew the shape of what needed tending.

My soon-to-be ex-husband showed up uninvited, unhinged, storming through the lobby of the very hotel we once owned together. Chaos followed him like smoke. I didn't see it coming. I never did. Sam found me alone, cracked open in the quiet, trying to steady my breath.

He didn't ask what happened. He didn't need to. He sat beside me and waited until I could look him in the eye.

"What is it you want most right now?" he asked.

I didn't hesitate. "To be free of this," I said. "I want my freedom."

He held my gaze, his voice low and deliberate. "Well then, what are you prepared to do for it?"

The question landed like a stone in water. No judgment. No urgency. Just the truth.

When the truth lands, you begin to understand that the life you live was shaped long before this moment. It attracted you to this relational dynamic and convinced you to stay long after its expiry date. My life was rooted deeply in a maternal history I hadn't dared to face.

Leaving him was supposed to feel liberating. Instead, I felt like I entered the gates of Hell and stared into a deep abyss with no safety net and no answers.

At the time, I didn't know Sam's question would become a lifelong threshold.

Freedom from what?

Not just from a relationship.

Not just from someone else's chaos.

But from the deeper patterns that kept me entangled: self-doubt, people-pleasing, and learned helplessness dressed in spiritual language.

Taking care of others was my kryptonite.

What followed wasn't a single, sweeping transformation. It was a quiet revolution.

Not the kind you announce to the world, but the kind that begins in a single room, when you finally realize something different is about to happen. A reckoning.

Not loud. Not linear. Not branded with certainty, but marked by a series of small, brave questions.

There was no map, just a feeling in my body—sometimes faint, sometimes fierce—that whispered, *What will you do for your freedom?* I had to learn to follow the answers. To live them over and over. And I had to find a way to stay in my body while I navigated this new terrain.

I had to create a space for radical honesty and personal ownership of that soulful whisper for freedom. I opened Pandora's box, and this started with naming the wound: codependence.

In my mind, *codependent* was a dirty word used in a group I didn't want to be a part of. It's a bitter pill to swallow, that moment you see yourself reflected in the very dynamic you spent years denying.

I spent my life in the personal development world. I knew the language of empowerment, self-responsibility, even boundaries. But when my marriage began to fall apart, I was confronted with a truth I wasn't ready to name. For all my strength and self-awareness, I built my life around managing others' emotional terrain—and my agency slipped quietly out the door I opened.

Codependence is a relational wound, but it's not just about unhealthy attachment. It's a form of internalized oppression. It teaches you to abandon yourself in the service of harmony, to confuse love with sacrifice, and to believe your worth is measured by your usefulness to others. Over time, this creates a quiet war inside: one part of you constantly performing, rescuing, proving, while the deeper, truer self is exiled.

It reveals itself in the push and pull of survival, in the anxious silence after someone's rage, in the way we contort ourselves to keep the peace. And it can wear many faces: spiritual, high functioning, even loving.

We become so skilled at reading the room, managing moods, and minimizing our own needs that we forget there was ever a self underneath.

It's a kind of disappearance.

What followed the rupture in that hotel room was one of the loneliest, most disorienting periods of my life. I didn't just lose a relationship—I lost the person I was inside of it. The version of me who kept things together, who took up just enough space to be acceptable, who knew how to survive by staying on the edge.

In the quiet that followed, I fell apart—not all at once, but in waves.

And yet, there was something else growing, too. Something slow. Something steady. Something I couldn't yet name and didn't know how to touch.

It lived beneath the noise of my doubt, beneath the ache and the unravelling, like a small flame protected from the wind, asking nothing of me but a quiet presence. On nights when I couldn't sleep, I imagined myself coming down a winding staircase to sit with this flame. It felt like a talisman; not something I carried in my hand, but something that lived inside me.

Around that time, I came across a line—its origin now lost to memory—that stirred a distant longing in me. It spoke of a place within untouched by trauma. I read those words over and over, unsure if I believed them. My body felt like a map of old wounds, each one etched into muscle and memory.

But whatever I imagined, this talisman took on a life of its own—not as a concept, but as a living, breathing, persistent truth.

A place within me that remained whole, unfettered; a quiet flame protected from the wind, marking the way back to myself. A place of remembering.

After years spent in unpredictable, chaotic environments—and even the well-intentioned noise of healing spaces where we jumped and shouted our way toward joy—I couldn't hear the sound of my voice, least of all the quiet one that rose from within.

The language of fixing and improving felt hollow, like rearranging furniture in a house with no foundation. What I was longing for wasn't another strategy; it was a deeper kind of restoration.

And I needed a different kind of listening—one that supported internal reclamation and could hold the weight of what I uncovered. I no longer sought self-improvement; I sought self-intimacy. I wanted a relationship with this deeper part of myself.

And I had no map for this kind of journey.

So, I had to create one—one that wasn't about progress but presence. Self-intimacy meant turning toward myself with the kind of attention I long reserved for others. It was learning to stay with my sensations, needs, and emotions without trying to fix or flee them; not performing wholeness but witnessing what was raw, tender, and real.

And at first, this was so uncomfortable.

My therapist gently suggested meditation, but the idea of sitting still felt impossible. It wasn't just uncomfortable; it felt unreachable, like a language I hadn't yet learned. And while my intellect understood the merits, my body was too charged, too alert. Stillness felt dangerous, not healing.

My body was a temple of hypervigilance, sacred only in its devotion to survival. On the outside, I appeared calm and composed. But just beneath the surface, a quiet storm churned. It was like trying to meditate inside a pressure cooker: thoughts ricocheting, breath shallow, muscles coiled tight, as if bracing for an impact that never came.

Stillness didn't feel like peace; it felt like exposure, like all the alarms I silenced suddenly rang at once. The quake was internal, invisible, but constant—a nervous system shaped by years of alertness, now struggling to trust the absence of threat.

So, I asked for help—a quiet prayer to an unknown source.

I need a practice to hold me. Something gentle. Please.

THE TOOL

Shortly after, in the quiet ache of early dawn, a whisper rose from the flame within me—a remembering of a practice I once witnessed a few years before my marriage ended. It waited patiently, this flicker of knowing, until I was still enough to feel its warmth.

What about qigong?

One of my earliest encounters with qigong (chee kung), a form of meditative movement, came during my final year of undergraduate studies while I was interning at a healing institute. A Japanese artist sought treatment for a terminal illness untouched by other methods. He brought only one person with him: his translator, who was also his qigong teacher.

Each morning, I watched from a distance as the artist moved through the courtyard, his body tracing shapes I didn't yet understand. There was no urgency in him, only presence. The gestures were slow and deliberate, like a language older than words. I remember the way his arms curved through the air, how his palms floated and turned, as if responding to something I couldn't see.

It was beautiful; it made my heart swell. I had never seen someone move like that—so tenderly, as if the body itself were a prayer. It broke something open in me. I felt a long breath leave my body. It was the kind of exhale that emptied centuries; a soft surrender that didn't ask for answers, only presence.

One day, I found the translator alone and asked him about the graceful form I saw. "It's qigong," he said simply.

I heard the term before, but something in the way he spoke invited deeper curiosity. "He seems so devoted to it," I remarked.

The translator replied, "It's not about curing his body," he said. "It's about how he meets his illness. Qigong teaches him to move with what is. It helps him have a better attitude."

I had no idea what a gift this would be.

Though that first encounter with qigong left a visceral imprint—an unmistakable sense of relief in my body—I wasn't yet ready to let it take root. Over the years, I picked it up and put it down like a book I couldn't quite finish, drawn to its wisdom but hesitant to let it fully shape me. I studied the form, learned its sequences, even taught parts of it, but some part of me held back.

Looking back now, I wonder if I was afraid—not of the practice itself, but of how profoundly it might change everything if I truly let it in. There's a strange ache in knowing something can nourish you, yet feeling unable to receive it. A lifetime of exile trained my body to turn away from the very thing it longed for.

Seven years passed since that first moment in the courtyard—seven years of shedding, unraveling, and slowly returning. And somewhere in that long undoing, I found myself reaching again for the practice I once held at a distance. Only this time, I didn't let go. What was once a curiosity became a lifeline, then a rhythm, then a home.

Qigong is no longer something I *do*; it's the scaffolding beneath everything, the quiet architecture of my being. It holds the shape of my days, my breath, my presence. It's the womb in which a new life gestated, the steady pulse beneath the surface of my becoming.

In the Taoist tradition, the force cultivated through qigong isn't push or pull; it's something quieter, more original. Like a stem cell, undifferentiated and unclaimed, it carries no fixed identity, no need to become anything at all. It enters the body not as a command, but as a whisper: pure potential.

I didn't always notice it at first. But slowly, as I returned to the same simple gestures each day, something began to shift. It was as if this neutral force slipped into me like light through a crack, finding its way into the places I armored. It didn't demand change. It just came, sensing, supporting, and softly rearranging.

Like a quiet hand on the small of my back, it knew where to go before I did. And wherever it moved, balance followed.

Through gentle, repetitive movements, we create enough spaciousness for the body's intelligence to rise. Spaciousness becomes the medicine. The true center of your being—the part untouched by trauma or identity—doesn't need to be built. It needs to be revealed.

As my devotion deepened, the outer forms of qigong began to open an inner door, one that led me into the subtle realms of Taoist inner alchemy. What began as movement through space evolved into movement through silence. Breath gave way to stillness, and stillness gave way to presence. I began to sense the inner landscape as a living cosmos, with elements, organs, and energies in sacred conversation.

And it gave me the "better attitude" the Japanese translator spoke of.

The freedom I sought began to take shape. No longer spinning in someone else's orbit, I became my own axis. This gave me the capacity to move through the relationship's death, with its many twists and turns, and to see my part in the evolution of a narrative I was ready to be free from.

I've tried many healing modalities over the years: therapy, retreats, somatic release, psychedelic work, spiritual intensives. Some offered moments of breakthrough, even brilliance. But more often than not, they left me disoriented, flooded with insight but without the inner scaffolding to hold it all—a place where these insights could become wisdom.

But in the still, spiraled rhythm of qigong movements, I found a space that could hold all of me.

It was something I could return to, again and again, not to escape the pain, but to stay present to it without leaving myself behind. And each time I practiced, I felt myself root even more deeply into the center: the center of my own being.

This journey inward was never just about energy or form; it was about finding a way back through the wound that first split me open. The rupture in that hotel room—the moment I realized how far I had drifted from myself—wasn't just a breaking, but a summons, a relational wound that could only be healed through relationship. Through the practices of qigong and Taoist inner alchemy, I've come to know a self intimacy that doesn't take, rescue, or abandon, but listens, restores, and remains.

What I've shared here is simply my understanding of this rich inner tradition as I know it *today*. This work continues to shape me as much as I shape it. Through these practices, I remain in conversation with my body, with the Tao, and with the many teachers and lineages that offered their wisdom along the way.

This is not a doctrine. It's a living path from rupture to restoration, from reaching outward to returning inward. And the more I walk it, the more I see how healing isn't about becoming perfect; it's about becoming *relational* with the self, with the body, and with the deeper rhythm that lives beneath the noise.

And while no single practice can heal everything, some open the door. So, I'll leave you with one: simple, subtle, and quietly powerful. It's called the Inner Smile. A practice of intention. A declaration of choosing yourself.

The Inner Smile is a foundational practice rooted in ancient Taoist inner alchemy. Originating from early Taoist sages who observed nature as the ultimate teacher, the practice was developed as a way to cultivate harmony within the body by directing loving awareness inward.

I hope it meets you where you are.

PRACTICE: THE INNER SMILE

Find a quiet place. Sit comfortably and close your eyes. Bring your awareness to your face and gently smile—not a forced grin, but a soft, inward gesture of warmth. Let this smile travel down into your eyes, your jaw, and your throat. Then guide it to your heart and pause. Feel your heart receive the smile, as if a dear friend just arrived.

Continue down—lungs, liver, stomach, kidneys—offering each organ a gentle smile of appreciation. There's no need to fix or analyze. Just notice, soften, and smile. Let the body remember it's safe to be held from within.

The chapter you have just read is one thread woven into a larger tapestry: *The Bones of Love*, a body of work devoted to ethical embodiment and the slow, sacred work of becoming whole. If something stirred while reading, I invite you to stay curious. There's more to come—more stories, more practices, more ways of remembering how to return to yourself with integrity, tenderness, and truth.

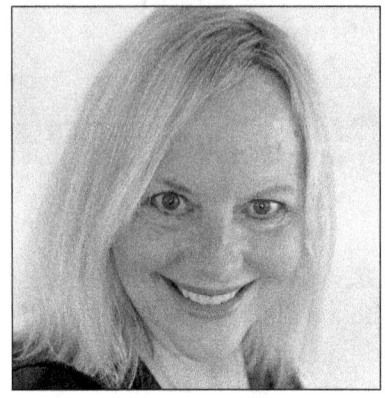

Laurie Cossar is not your typical guide; she's a quiet revolutionary.

Rooted in Taoist philosophy, trauma-informed practice, and the subtle language of the body, Laurie's work emerges from a lifetime of unravelling and remembering. After decades spent in personal development alongside leaders like Tony Robbins and the late Wayne Dyer, she discovered true freedom isn't in fixing, but in reclaiming the self from the grip of societal programming and codependent paradigms.

Through her writing and the sharing of gentle, embodied practices, Laurie offers a way back to what has never been lost: your inner authority. She helps readers recognize and release the unconscious agreements that keep them bound to old roles and invites them to design a life rooted in awareness, integrity, and choice.

A Taoist at heart, Laurie honors the cyclical rhythm of insight and rest. While her practices are spacious and gentle, they are also unafraid to enter the darker corridors of the self, the places where sovereignty was once surrendered. This is a path of disruption and tenderness, where discomfort becomes a doorway and each threshold is met with care. She doesn't promise to lead from the front, but instead to walk beside you quietly, fiercely, and with unwavering integrity.

Laurie's current body of work lives inside her forthcoming book, *The Bones of Love: The Ethical Embodiment of Our Spiritual Practice*, and a digital sanctuary in progress. Readers called to her story are invited to follow the thread, not toward her, but toward themselves.

If you feel called, you're welcome to reach out, whether for one-on-one support, guidance in your practice, or to stay close to this unfolding work.

Connect with Laurie:

Website: http://www.thebonesoflove.com/
Email: laurie@thebonesoflove.com

CHAPTER 7

Memories: Unknown, Lost, or Forgotten

How Our Wombs Experience Domestic Violence and Trauma

Ruby Raja

I dare you to imagine life without abuse.
~ Ruby Raja

MY STORY

Domestic violence can seriously harm unborn babies in the womb and can affect their lives in ways we can't imagine. Statistics tell us that trauma occurs in seven percent of all pregnancies (Mestaghinia, Sooky, and Mestaghinia 2012), and the most significant impact on the womb is that of intimate partner violence (IPV); in other words, domestic violence between a man and a woman.

Untreated womb trauma can be overwhelming, with the unborn child being at risk of becoming the adult who cannot manage their life because they simply don't understand what they're dealing with. The mother and unborn child should receive support from a place of love and kindness, including in any research.

My exposure to this phenomenon began in 2007 when I started working as a probation officer in England. The histories of my clients, known as *offenders*, clearly showed they hadn't received care in a meaningful way. It appeared most had parents who were either not there—maybe they were working—or their fathers abused their mothers. The offenses they committed were broad, and the number of domestic violence offenses was high and increasing.

I didn't realize where my journey in the criminal justice system would take me. I worked with men, women, and children experiencing domestic violence for decades, sometimes not even knowing it, because I worked voluntarily, helping anyone I could. They shared their deepest, most intimate secrets with me, but I never recorded anything–a gift I realized much later was critical in protecting victims from the abuse that legal professionals and court systems put them through.

Entering the world of justice would be a conflict I had to survive if I were to share my story.

I believed the men and women on probation whom I managed were not criminals. My clients were born into a world of chaos, pain, neglect, abuse, domestic violence, and sexual abuse. More importantly, no one cared for or listened to them. Few received any fragments of the love and care we assume all babies and children receive unconditionally.

My journey of understanding what happens in the womb began here—so I thought. It was directly related to domestic violence and its impact on mothers and, by default, the unborn. I held this profound belief and I remember feeling very lonely with this idea. No one else uttered such thoughts.

Is it only me who thinks that clients are not criminals and their trauma begins in the womb?

I remembered a few years earlier, while delivering domestic violence training to frontline practitioners, I was asked, "How do you work with a woman who's carrying a baby, but the baby has died due to extreme violence from her partner?" This was at a time when the UK was in its early days of exploring domestic violence.

MY OWN WOMB TRAUMA: UNKNOWN, LOST, OR FORGOTTEN

I began my journey into understanding domestic violence and womb trauma by observing patterns in many of my clients, which I believe originated in the womb. What I didn't yet know was where womb trauma truly stemmed from. I hadn't discovered my own "why."

In the mid-1990s, I suffered a miscarriage from which I healed well, due to a support and belief system that protects, guides, and nurtures me. I was surrounded by people who cared, dropping tiny little love bombs in the shape of gentle guidance. They shared their heartbreaks and experiences. Sharing grief and pain is a regular part of my experiences within the circles I'm a part of.

This type of sharing *can* be brutal.

I'd describe it as something that feels impossible but opens up a space you didn't think you needed. We tend not to make everything an issue, so it gives us time and space for thoughts ahead of where we are. It contradicts all Western standards, as it's not always about *me*. It's often about finding ourselves in places we didn't know about—some places infringing on what the West says are our rights, which I believe fractures our ability to go beyond and into the future.

When I raised my children, I practiced giving them unspoken permission to explore. I gave them a little more than they needed because I knew they would need it. Life feels less frightening when a door or window is opened for you and you've been given permission to explore. You can choose whether to peek through, walk through, or even just keep opening and closing until you feel safe enough to make your move.

A feeling of safety is created for you, and you don't even know it. From that safety comes empowerment, and from a place of empowerment, you can make better decisions for yourself. It's this aspect that enables you to believe and start moving out of the space others have created for you into the real you, and that's where I'd like to take you, to finding your true self.

My personal experience of womb trauma felt like this:

"You already have a son and a daughter; what more do you want? You need to have a hysterectomy now." These were the words my second OB-GYN hurled at me as she demanded the right to take my uterus. Having just miscarried, I was in a state of confusion, shock, and trauma.

This was not the first time my second OB-GYN was unprofessional and unkind. She seemed to own and take rights she didn't have, like insisting I needed a hysterectomy. Compassionate professions require humanity, dignity, sensitivity, and kindness. These words were not in her vocabulary. She didn't see me; she saw the dollars she could make, a true patriot of the US pharmaceutical and medical industry.

She matters little to me, as does her opinion.

It was only on reflection that I realized how fortunate I was to feel secure with my opinions about her. We assume a professional's words are set in stone. After all, she was the doctor, and I had little understanding of what losing a baby looked like medically. Neither did I understand the alleged moral, ethical, financial, and other value judgments. That was her field.

When someone directs you to do something, DON'T DO IT. Stop, reflect, question, and know you are always the most important person in the situation.

I knew a series of steps were required before serious actions were taken, but evil has no bounds. She didn't even consider a blood test, which is all it took for me to find out I had an underactive thyroid. One tablet would balance the imbalance that led to my miscarriage, and here she stood, telling me my uterus needed to be removed—*taken* from me.

Imagine all the things that could have gone wrong if I listened to her. My mental health, first and foremost.

YOUNG PEOPLE

My work with young people triggered a deep wound within me; I didn't recognize it was as close to the surface as it is. Working with my clients brought it to the fore. It's easy to identify a trait in someone else, but how can we recognize our wound? It's painful, it hurts, and it's easier to ignore, to run away from, or to not deal with altogether.

Wrong.

It wasn't a painful journey; it was strangely familiar.

My clients themselves didn't trigger me. I was sad they didn't stand a chance because they would never know. How could they? I only knew because I was raised to question and to know I had rights, despite the West controlling people's narratives through the media.

MY WOMB TRAUMA EXPLAINED

I knew that when my first OB-GYN, a white American female, had done wrong, I still had rights. My then-husband didn't allow me to exercise those rights, but I knew the mistake was hers, not mine. This will remain an unresolved trauma as my then-husband would not allow me to pursue any course of action.

My first OB-GYN made a grave error in judgment, saying I was never pregnant, having confirmed my pregnancy less than a month earlier. She said, I'd had a 'missed' pregnancy which resulted in a D&C (dilation and curettage). Six weeks later, I had contractions for nearly seven days, and the contractions became more intense each day. It is strange to have contractions when there was no baby, and a D&C had taken place.

To add insult to injury, she did not return my calls, and I had to find a second OB-GYN to deal with what had happened. A 'missed' pregnancy was her professional stance.

I mourned this pregnancy twice because of an incompetent medical professional who lacked the decency to return my calls and deal with the problem she had created.

I shared earlier that I knew I had rights. I didn't know or understand what a missed pregnancy was. I didn't stop to question this. I bear the wounds of her ignorance and incompetence.

Once the second OB-GYN removed the fetus, I felt as though I was a woman again.

That sense of release ultimately set me free. It was a gateway to profound healing, which gave me tremendous insight into my own trauma, as well as that of my clients. Feeling whole again and desiring my client group to feel whole propelled me forward.

Returning to my work, I worked with 13-year-old girls who used violence toward their parents and grandparents. They were dream students according to all staff, from teachers to mentors, year heads to head-teachers. What made them strike out at 13 and 14 years of age?

Probation taught me to question every area of life, so I explored with professionals and took a deep dive into the girls' histories. The magic happened when I asked their mothers about their early childhood. Nothing of significance emerged, and then, I asked about pregnancy.

The arrow left the bow.

I asked simple questions about their pregnancy: 'What was your pregnancy like? Did you work? Were you sick in the early stages?' These questions led to disclosures of being with an abuser.

"It wasn't as much the pregnancy as my husband/partner I was with. It became too much."

Most mums didn't know they were experiencing domestic violence in the womb, but all were with abusers.

One mum told me she left her partner in the sixth month of her pregnancy and never wanted to talk about it ever again.

Kudos!

Great news, except that her daughter will never know why she has rage and what triggers it. Her daughter will live her life being exceptional, but with a rage that explodes—or will she?

This case led me to dig deeper and explore wider. I worked with women and men who experienced domestic violence. I could see their child or children were affected in ways they could never understand. I was powerless to do anything officially, but that didn't mean I couldn't gather my own evidence and knowledge and experientially begin my own safe testing of options for babies born through trauma as a result of domestic violence.

That's what I decided to do.

I recognized that knowing you've experienced domestic violence doesn't mean you know or understand how to manage it. I created a program that doesn't tell people what to do; it allows them to explore, think, take, or leave what I open up for them, and make sense of their own world.

What's critical about the program is that it provides tools and explains how domestic violence works. Then you can question and challenge yourself in ways you couldn't imagine. It permits you to know, to understand, to be, to *unleash the real you.*

To begin this intense and intimate journey, you need someone you can trust who understands the delicate balance of care necessary to heal from such trauma.

What I've shared is as intense as it is intimate.

THE TOOL

DEFINE YOURSELF! (DY!) PROGRAM

I authored *Healing from Narcissistic Abuse–Journeys from Abuse to Freedom* (2025) when participants from my master's thesis, *How Women Escape the Self-Imposed Controls of Marriage (2017),* told me they became fully independent using information I gave them. They were able to explain coercive control and narcissistic behaviors to their lawyers and use other information in court to safeguard their children.

I created Define Yourself! because I believed that if women became fully independent of their abusers in two and a half years using my guidance, this program needed to be made available for everyone. People need to be kinder to themselves and know they can set themselves free by breaking the chains that control them. I can see how amazing people are, and by changing the lens they view life from, they too can live full, independent lives, free of the abuse they've experienced.

With Define Yourself!, you become the focus of your life, and find the amazing person hidden within, you find out who you truly are. You'll understand how patriarchy, culture, and religion affect your life and the decisions you make.

By understanding your thoughts on what you can or can't do according to your belief and value system, you'll be able to permit yourself to behave in a way that until now, you may have believed to be wrong.

What I found with the participants of my book was that they were crippled until they learned they weren't doing anything against their Lord or clergy, and they weren't being disobedient to their parents. Most importantly, they realized their wonderful mothers and friends, whilst fully supportive of them, did not and could not understand the dynamics of domestic violence. This small, all-encompassing fact—*power and control* by an intimate partner—if not understood, can cause untold damage inadvertently, in the healing process.

Victims need to understand this fact, and any practitioner who can enable people to make their own decisions is gold dust. Many practitioners are taught to tick boxes, which often involves telling people what to do.

Once applied to your own life, you'll have flickers of light and connections, followed by full-blown, "I knew I wasn't crazy, it really was happening to me the way I thought," moments.

Reclaim your life with Define Yourself!

The world is waiting for you.

A SIMPLE REFLECTION EXERCISE

So many internal conflicts arise not from reality, but from a belief system passed down or imposed. A simple reflection exercise to try Define Yourself! in your own way might look like this:

Ask yourself:

- What do I believe I "can't" do—and why?
- Who told me that was wrong?
- Why can't I do it?
- What would I do differently if I gave myself permission?

By naming these inherited beliefs, we begin to loosen their grip. You are not disobedient. You are awakening.

Carl Jung reminds us: "Who looks outside, dreams; who looks inside, awakens." (Jung, 1965).

And Rumi offers us: "The wound is where the light enters you." (Good Vibe Quotes.)

Let this light guide you.

Use that wound and make it your reason to Define Yourself! A whole new world awaits you when you make your decision.

And now, I invite you to close your eyes and imagine with me.

You've made a decision to define yourself on your own terms. What might that look and feel like in six months?

You've begun shifting your beliefs, reclaiming your autonomy, and finding joy in the mirror again.

What do you see?

Who are you becoming?

What might the world feel like when you're finally free?

Isn't it beautiful? Perhaps a little scary?

I invite you to take the first step; it's the one that will set you free.

Please open your eyes and feel what it felt like.

When we speak about the womb, we have to realise that healing the womb is not an abstract issue. I've begun collecting stories and data from women who have experienced trauma in utero or while pregnant, often under unimaginable conditions. Not only are these stories sacred, but healing can only take place by hearing these stories.

Healing is taking place, but not enough people know about it.

Your story matters. Even if you forget, your body remembers (VdK, 2014, www.inshiraa.com/resources/books), it keeps the score. Your healing will set you free and release future generations from the pain you carry.

I'm currently documenting one such journey, of a woman who survived extreme domestic violence and abuse during multiple pregnancies and is now thriving, despite being failed by the U.S. justice system. Her story, and others like it, will help illuminate the path forward. I'd like to invite you to visit: www.inshiraa.com and https://YouTube/@inshiraa-ruby where new information will be released.

REFERENCES:

Jung, C. G., & Jaffé, A. (1965). Memories, dreams, reflections. Rev. ed. Vintage Books.

Mesdaghinia E, Sooky Z, Mesdaghinia A. "Causes of trauma in pregnant women referred to Shabih-Khani Maternity Hospital in Kashan." *Arch Trauma Res.* 2012 Spring;1(1):23-6. doi: 10.5812/atr.5291. Epub 2012 Jun 1. PMID: 24719837; PMCID: PMC3955936.

Raja, R. (2017). MSc Thesis. "How Women Escape the Self-Imposed Controls of Marriage," Bristol. (Unpublished but accessible through www.inshiraa.com.)

Raja, R. (2025). *Healing from Narcissistic Abuse–Journeys from Abuse to Freedom.* London.

Rumi. (N.d.) Good Vibe Quotes; 85 Inspirational Rumi Quotes on Love. Accessedon 7th July 2025, https://inspiregoodvibes.com/blogs/news/rumi-quotes-love-inspirational

Van der Kolk, B. A. (2014). The Body Keeps the Score: Brain, Mind, and Body in the Healing of Trauma. Viking.

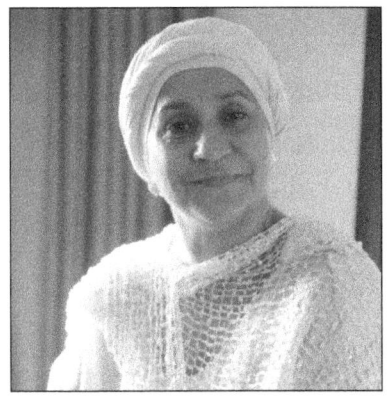

Ruby Raja, DipPS, MSc, is the Founder of Inshiraa, a website for people experiencing domestic violence and trauma. She's the author of *Healing from Narcissistic Abuse—Journeys from Abuse to Freedom* and writes for *Her Nation*, an online magazine for women.

Ruby partners with organisations in London and delivers domestic violence and trauma services to men, women, and children. She works with schools, places of worship, and individuals.

Ruby partners with an organisation in the USA/Costa Rica where they deliver domestic violence and trauma services online and are planning retreats in the USA.

Ruby began exploring the field of trauma after being attacked next to the House of Commons in London while on her morning walk. She became a Certified Trauma Facilitator and Trainer (ACCPH) for the BeyondTrauma Academy and delivers specialised trauma services for practitioners to be truly trauma-informed in their workplace and for victims to heal from trauma.

She believes victims of attack must learn to trust themselves and not be swayed by so-called professionals, especially prosecutors and the court system, and they must never change their narrative. The true picture of trauma emerges when your mind and body feel safe and relaxed, and that takes time.

Ruby's most ardent desire is to help keep families who experience abuse safe and together, where realistic, by empowering them to reclaim their lives after abuse, especially precious newborn babies.

Connect with Ruby:

Website: http://www.inshiraa.com

LinkedIn: https://www.linkedin.com/in/ruby-raja-681908302/

Email: info.inshiraa@gmail.com

YouTube: YouTube.com/@inshiraa-ruby

You can find *Healing from Narcissistic Abuse–Journeys from Abuse to Freedom* at: www.inshiraa.com/my-book

CHAPTER 8

Birthing Magic

Being Divinely Supported by Your Guides

Mandy Webb Hancock, CD, PCD, CBE

MY STORY

"No," I said as the tears welled up. "No!"

This time, my voice cracked as I started to sob inconsolably.

How the hell does a birth plan get so derailed when I've done everything right?!

I looked around at the cold, sterile hospital room. The fluorescent lights stung my eyes. Or was that the salty tears? A combination, no doubt.

The blanket draped over my legs felt like sandpaper. It smelled like bleach. The monitor surrounding my 39-weeks-and-four-days belly felt like a ball and chain, forcing me to stay on the uncomfortably thin mattress. I looked down at the blood pressure cuff as it tightened again, crushing my arm for the umpteenth time that evening. They had me tethered to the bed.

I couldn't leave if I wanted to. My thoughts raced.

My pink jacket hung on the lone chair in the corner of the room. It was the only thing there that wasn't white or grey.

I wallowed to myself. *This feels like a prison.*

I whimpered as my husband grabbed my hand and squeezed, with a fear in his eyes I hadn't seen before.

With a wife who's a childbirth educator as well as a birth and bereavement doula, he was well aware of the statistical dangers of a hospital birth. He knew why I was so shaken. And I could see by the way he fidgeted that he was just as unsure as I was about this change of plans.

"Mandy, your blood pressure is fluctuating, and it's hitting possible stroke levels. We need the baby to come now." The nurse was empathetic, but this was not what we wanted to hear.

My first baby was born at a birth center: the second, a beautiful and peaceful home birth.

That's what I wanted this time, too. That's what we prepared for. We rented the birth tub, bought the birth kit, paid off the entire out-of-pocket invoice for the midwife, took the refresher birthing course, made the playlist, bought all the perfect labor snacks, everything.

At one of our prenatal appointments, I asked my midwife if she thought he'd be born late, like the first two. "Third babies are a wildcard," she said. And now this.

A wildcard, indeed.

The obstetrician was kind enough and allowed us to go home for a few hours to at least put a bag of essentials together and make arrangements for our two older children. We'd come back shortly. I had to be induced.

I stared out the car window, the glow of the passing vehicles and streetlights a blur. I was distraught. I took a deep breath in, unable to keep it from being audibly shaky.

"Babe, it's all going to be okay." My sweet husband treaded lightly as he attempted to reassure me.

We pulled into the driveway and my best friend met us at the door. "How do I do this?" I wept to her when we arrived. "I'm terrified!"

Saying the words out loud made it even more real, and at that moment, the pregnancy hormones kicked into overdrive. I had another cathartic cry; thankful the kids were already asleep.

She held my hands in hers and leaned in. "Mandy, I know this isn't what you planned. But you have the strength of all the women before you and the body, mind, and spirit wisdom of Source energy. You know that God/Goddess has got this. You can do *anything* with that kind of support. Hell, this could be your best birth yet."

That last part of her comment shifted something in me.

Could it?

I already painted this experience as something horrible, something to be feared. But it hadn't even happened yet, and in that moment, I remembered one of my favorite quotes by Mark Twain: "I've had a lot of worries in my life, most of which never happened."

I felt a warm rush of peace wash over me. She was right. *Maybe this could be my best birth yet.* Of course, my emotions were running high, and I *was* devastated, but deep down, I knew I could do it. I'd had two babies naturally, unmedicated. If I could do that, I could do anything, anywhere, especially with the power of God behind and within me.

Even if the hospital setting seemed entirely counterintuitive to the natural process of birth, and some of the things I saw as a birth worker had me very distrustful of the whole system, I just risked out of my planned home birth. And gestational hypertension was not something to mess around with. It was a medically necessary transfer of care. Simple as that. Still, it sucked.

I took a slow, deliberate breath in and blew it out through pursed lips. Time to accept the new plan and recalibrate with the divine help of Great Spirit.

The induction went as smoothly as it could. Once I realized the potential of this experience, I could go in with a clear head and a readiness that felt brave and courageous. I knew how to advocate for myself and that I would have an amazing birth, despite the change in circumstances.

My body was ready, and all the interventions were successful.

I was "in the zone." Childbirth is this incredibly fascinating process where mama must go inward to bring her baby outward. It's an insanely physical job. They don't call it "labor" for nothing.

But it's just as much of a mind game as it is body. And at some point, the spirit must get involved as well. It's the holy trinity of help to get a mother past that finish line. It requires the mind, body, and spirit, in unison, for birth to triumphantly happen. And during this miraculous journey, the veil is *thin*.

I knew this to be the case from my previous two births, as well as other births I witnessed. There's always a moment, usually during transition, where the mother is so exhausted and the sensations so intense that she thinks she can't do it.

She's beyond tired. The crashing waves of contractions take her to the edge of existence. She's been swimming against the current for too long, and now, she feels like she's drowning.

This is a transition in birth. This brief but severe period that comes right before the birth of the baby is the epitome moment when wild nature takes over and the mind, body, and spirit show up together to carry out this indescribably monumental task.

It's when the body has been working so hard to bring the baby down and out of the sacred womb space, and into the portal that will eventually lead to life on Earth.

Every contraction requires immense energy, and it feels like there's just none left. The baby enters the birth canal, and the astronomical amount of pressure is overwhelming.

The thread between life and death in childbirth is ever so delicate. Push it too far, and it can snap. A birthing mother walks this line like a tightrope.

This is where the mama thinks she can't. And this is where I was, in that frigid and vacant hospital room, when I internally called out to God: *I can't do this. Help me!*

In that instant, something amazing happened. Suddenly, the insufferable anguish subsided, and I was floating in space. The tribulation paused, and a profound sense of support and nurturance met me.

My gaze traveled upward, and I beheld a brilliant and luminous white light that poured toward me, overcoming any other feeling I had besides pure, powerful, vibrant **love**.

I slowly distinguished a line of women, one by one, who appeared in the gleaming pillar of light. Each one stair-stepped in descending succession from the abundant glow, all the way down to me.

Their presence was familiar. Intimate. Comforting. Even though I didn't recognize the ones at the top from this lifetime, I knew immediately these souls were those of my ancestors, guides, and guardian angels.

Another burst of radiance appeared, and I watched as a tiny baby—my baby—passed from the immaculate Source energy light to the first divine female presence in the expansive column of illuminated queens.

She whispered something sweet in the baby's ear, tenderly kissed his cheek, then gently handed him to the next stunning member of this supernatural counsel.

The second goddess lovingly hugged him, whispered another precious sentiment, softly kissed his forehead, and compassionately passed him to the subsequent light being in the quintessential and immortal line.

This went on and on, ever so slowly and deliberately, with exceptional care.

As my child came closer, I recognized the ethereal woman. My great-grandmother, whom I knew and loved until she passed when I was 17, told me telepathically, "I am so proud of you. I am always with you, guiding you."

My grandmother was next. I never met her, as she died before I was born, but I saw her in many family photos. In the same way, speaking with the mind, she let me know she'd been watching me and supporting me since I was an egg in my own mother, while *my* mom was being shaped in *her* womb. The genetic connection to our ancestors spans over multiple generations. We are all interconnected.

I saw my best friend, who tragically passed away on my fifteenth birthday.

I frequently thought about this dear friend and how she was robbed of a life past her youth. I was oftentimes mournful and heartsick over the fact that she'd never be a mother—something she always wanted, even as a kid.

She was the one who made the final handoff. She was the woman bestowed with the gift of giving me my baby.

She looked at me through my eyes and down into my soul. She was joyfully honored to have undertaken this mission, and while bending time and space, she told me with a soft grin, "Do not grieve my 'loss', but cherish your life and your children for me and every other woman who wanted a child but never had one. But most of all, adore your own life, for you."

With a glint in her smile, she fulfilled her righteous duty. The crowning delivery of my baby from God was perfectly executed as she placed him in my awaiting arms.

With that cosmic action, I was jolted back into this dimension. With a powerful lioness roar and the strength and wisdom of every woman before me, I laid my hands on my baby as I transported him from my body, and from the infinite, Earthside.

It's a renowned fact that childbirth changes a person.

It's walking through the valley of the shadow of death, with the promised land at the end of the long, treacherous road. It's an intermingling of radical trust in the Divine and in your own ability to bring a child from the astral plane and into this realm. It's treading through hell to get to heaven on earth.

Birth is so symbolic of life in general. Many times, we go through different types of rebirths throughout our lifetime. We experience transcendental traumas and parts of us die, while what remains is reborn into a new version of ourselves.

Like a phoenix from the ashes, we rise anew.

Babies aren't the only things to be born from us, either. We shape ideas within and bring them into this density through labor and life transitions. Dreams are built internally until we go through the motions required to bring them to fruition.

This metaphysical journey reshaped my entire existence. What my great-grandmother said in that space between, soaring in the cosmos and grounded in reality, replayed in my head. She said, "I'm always with you, guiding you." What did that mean? Did it mean I could access her mystic wisdom and divine guidance at any time? Something inside me rang like a bell with a resounding *yes*.

But *how*?

THE TOOL

Once I came up for air after having this out-of-body adventure and officially becoming a family of five, I dove into studying and learning the ways I could tap into the magical space where this superior guidance and support were so readily available.

Turns out that communing with God and our guides is ancient medicine and practice. And somewhere down the road, we lost this unbreakable connection. We forgot.

My obsession with reestablishing this communicative ability led me down a path of metamorphosis. I was no longer separated from this area after opening the floodgates at birth. The more I read, trained, refined, and practiced, the easier it became.

I gained, or should I say, remembered, psychic capabilities. I went back to school and earned certifications as an intuitive psychic and healer. I studied and achieved credentials on how to facilitate breathwork.

I now use these skills with proficient mastery to help others through birth and rebirth.

Whether it be a physical birth of their baby or a rebirthing of a new version of themselves, I doula babies from womb to world, and I doula ideas from mind to reality.

Connecting with ancestors, guides, or angels can be a deeply personal and spiritual experience. Several methods can accelerate these connections. It's my greatest honor to share a few of my preferred methods with you here, starting with my personal favorite: a simple, guided meditation.

1. MEDITATION

Guided visualization:

- Find a quiet space where you won't be disturbed.
- Sit or lie down comfortably and close your eyes.
- Take several deep breaths, inhaling through your nose and exhaling through your mouth, allowing yourself to relax.

- Visualize a beautiful, bright light around you that represents protection and love. Nothing can enter this safe and secure sphere that isn't of the highest vibrational frequency.

- Imagine a staircase or path leading up into the sky and beyond. As you ascend, feel yourself getting lighter and more connected to the heavenly realms.

- Go above the atmosphere where space opens to the cosmos.

- Once you are there and have reached the top of your celestial staircase, call upon your ancestors, spirit guides, and angels. Speak to them in your mind or out loud, asking for guidance or communication. Get to know them by name.

- They can be in the form of light, animal spirit, totem, human, or other. You may recognize them as family or friends who've crossed over, like your grandma or best friend. They may be characters or beings you've only heard of, like Archangel Michael, Mary Magdalene, a medicine woman, or a warrior.

- You can call out to God, Buddha, or Yeshua. Source energy is always there, always available.

- Be open to any messages or feelings that come through, trusting your intuition.

- Take time here to be present for what is revealed. Take time to integrate what is shown.

- When you're ready to return, thank your guides for their wisdom and visualize descending the staircase, bringing back any insights gained during the experience and leaving what no longer serves you to be transmuted.

2. DREAM WORK

Before going to sleep, set an intention to connect with your ancestors or guides. Keep a dream journal to record any messages or symbols that appear in your dreams, as they can provide valuable insights.

3. MEDITATIVE JOURNEYING

This technique involves using rhythmic music or drumming to enter an altered state of consciousness. You can set an intention to meet your guides or ancestors and let the sound carry you into the multiverse. Transformative breathwork is amazing for this.

4. NATURE CONNECTION

Spend time in nature, where the energy is often more grounded and aligned with the spirit world. Listen to the whispers of the wind and allow nature to guide you in connecting with the Divine.

5. CEREMONIAL PRACTICES

Create a small altar with photographs or symbols representing your ancestors. Light candles and incense, and pray or meditate in front of the altar, inviting their presence into your space. Always remember to stay grounded and protected with your encompassing circle of light.

6. CHANNELING

Train yourself to channel messages by quieting your mind and allowing thoughts and words to flow freely. You might want to use free writing or recorded speaking to express the messages you receive.

7. USING TOOLS

Tools such as tarot cards, pendulums, or crystals can help you open a connection. Choose one that resonates with you and focus on your intention to communicate with elevated spirit guides, continually recalling grounding and protection when doing this work.

8. AFFIRMATIONS AND INTENTIONS

Use positive affirmations to call upon your ancestors or guides daily. Phrases like "I am open to receiving guidance from my ancestors" can create a space for connection in the macrocosm.

Each of these methods can be tailored to suit your personal beliefs and energy. Consistency and openness are key to deepening these connections, as is trusting your own intuition and the messages you may receive.

We all have the gift of this transcendental kinship. Our affinity for correspondence with our ancestors, guides, and angels goes beyond all time and space. There's a great remembering happening right now, and you're reading this book for a profound reason.

We're all connected, linked by the golden, familial thread of life that flows between this dimension and the rest. Never forget we're all one in the end, and that all beings are unconditionally loved and supported by Source, without exception, always, in all ways.

All my love to you, dear reader.

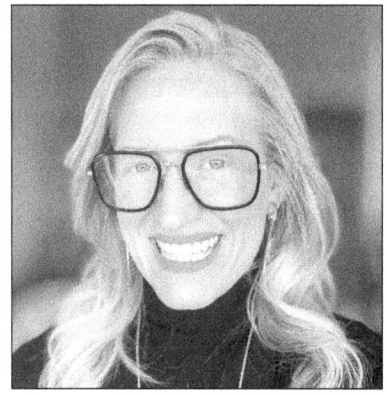

Mandy Webb Hancock is a joyfully busy working and homeschooling mom of four beautiful children, dedicated to enhancing others' lives through diverse talents and deep-rooted passions.

Mandy is an expert in numerous facets, with a calling for service. As the owner of multiple heart-led businesses, she wears many hats in her professional life.

Her impressive list of credentials includes roles as a full-spectrum, trauma-informed birth, postpartum, bereavement, and death doula; birth patient advocate; childbirth educator; birth trauma processing guide; digital entrepreneur and mentor; water priestess; transformational breathwork facilitator; intuitive psychic and healer; energetic worker; and ordained minister. She's an equal rights activist, author, artist, hair stylist, salon owner, and a passionate advocate for sustainability and peace.

Mandy believes in the transformative power of unity and collective consciousness. She envisions a world where people coexist harmoniously, emphasizing, "In this new paradigm, our goal is to rise together. There's room for all of us. There's more than enough for everyone." She recognizes that each individual is born with unique gifts essential for the world's tapestry.

Mandy is committed to fostering an environment where everyone feels valued and empowered. She understands the urgency of the shift toward peace. She's dedicated to being an active participant in this crucial journey.

Through her work and personal philosophy, Mandy inspires those around her to recognize their inherent worth and contribution to the greater good.

As a mother, advocate, and healer, Mandy is not just shaping her family's future; she's also actively working to create a brighter, more inclusive world for generations to come.

Connect with Mandy:

Website: https://www.blissfulbirth.co

Facebook: https://www.facebook.com/earthtomandy
https://www.facebook.com/blissfulbirth.co

Instagram: https://www.instagram.com/earthtomandy/

Birth Processing Workbook: https://a.co/d/4makgD3

CHAPTER 9

Becoming Possible

Finding Purpose Through Suicidality

Silen Wellington

Content note:
This chapter contains references to a suicide attempt and self-harm.

MY STORY

I'm 18 years old, and I've decided it's the perfect night to die.

It's a Colorado spring night in 2014. The asphalt is still warm from the sun, and a fresh cold curls around the dusk blue mountains.

I just finished playing piano with the swing band at my high school dance, my fingers electric from twisting over blues scales.

I'm parked on the side of a neighborhood with no sidewalks, on the edge of town, where the cottonwood trees click their fresh leaves together in greeting.

It's a perfect night to die, I keep singing in my head.

I leave my shoes in the car, kicking up loose rocks jutting out of the pavement where the road meets gravel. Then, gravel meets pine needles and grass, my feet treading a map I've walked many times before, until

I reach the silver beams of the railroad tracks, elevated on a long bed of rocks extending as far south as I can see.

My heart rate slows as soon as I see them.

It's a perfect night to die.

I step onto the beam, fix my eyes on the star ahead, low on the horizon, and walk.

Time loosens, shifts into lungs that expand and contract, matching my breath with the precarity of my bare feet on a silver beam. Normally, I'm scared of night, but here, I'm calm, feeling the warmth of escaping it all.

Suddenly, the clouds rustle and light up. The wind blows my hair in every direction. I bend my knees, ducking my head as I keep walking, sliding over the beam against the new spring gusts.

And then, the lightning strikes.

So close, it blurs my vision.

And again—

I see nothing but the brightness of it—no hills, no tracks, just light.

Have I already died?

The night shadows come back into focus until the next flash of lightning, as bright as the first, blazes eternity across my vision.

The wind screeches. I listen to the storm, the thunderclaps breaking the sky, a far-off whistle. The light beckons me to become one with the world.

You can't stay here.

It isn't my own voice—or at least, not a voice I recognize—but it arises from within me.

My body wants to sink into the wooden planks, to become damp and decayed, but the storm is screaming, *Leave.*

It's not my night to die.

Leave!

I turn around, wind gripping my face and toes blistering against the rocks between the railroad tracks.

I'm heaving when I make it back to my car, my clothes soaked.

Something courses through me, like someone plugged an electrical charge into me. It's flowing up and down my arms, making me vibrate like a cello string.

* * *

When I was growing up, I didn't feel *possible*. By possible, I don't mean possibility—my life was brimming with possibility. I grew up in Colorado, upper middle class, white, in the kind of suburban dream that included piano lessons and water fights in the park with my friends.

But still, something felt deeply wrong. And by that, I mean I couldn't see myself living for very long.

For almost a decade, we—me, my friends, and the adults around me—weren't really sure if I was going to live or die.

I went to therapy off and on for seven years and tried various psychiatric medications. But even after seven years of those things, I didn't see myself belonging to the world. I needed something else; I needed to find community, discover who I was, and find spaces where I could be celebrated for who I was.

* * *

It's summer 2014. I'm at a therapeutic rite of passage dance camp for youth.

I arrive here in part through serendipity, and in part through desperation. I'm desperate to try anything but the medication that numbed my senses and made me lightheaded.

The first day of camp, I'm paired with a young man named Robin with long blonde hair, and the kind of smile that radiates love. We take turns tracing each other's bodies on paper so we can fill them in with our stories through drawings and collage.

When it's time to trace my body, I lie down in something like a fetal position, my limbs reaching out, as if I've collapsed on a set of railroad tracks. I'm wearing a green dress that usually falls to my knees, but when I lie down, it lifts up, revealing the angry purple scars on my legs—*battle scars*, my friends and I have come to call them. I close my eyes and stiffen as I feel Robin's purple marker trace around my legs, anticipating the inevitable question I don't want to answer.

Thankfully, he doesn't ask.

Later, we end up at the same host family's house, talking for hours about art and how we decided to arrive at this summer camp. Then, in the quiet after midnight, Robin looks me in the eye, gestures to my exposed thighs, and says:

"So, tell me about this art."

It's the most generous, gracious, and understanding way anyone has ever asked about my self-harm scars. I've been stared at. I've been pointed at. I've been asked in shocked voices. I've been asked in blatantly disgusted voices. *What the fuck happened to your legs?* I've been asked with smirks that knew the answer before the question, smirks that just wanted to hear how I'd lie about it. I've been asked with quiet horror.

Never had I been asked with the intention to know more about the beautiful parts of me. *So, tell me about this art.*

* * *

I didn't realize it at the time, but my spirit hadn't decided to fully be here. The storm called me back, and I needed an initiation.

I was in the rhythm of chaos, the rumbling, rag-dolled, breaking-open-on-the-drumhead dance of, *Who am I?* And, *Why am I?*

My spirit needed to decide to step into adulthood and get acquainted with the unique gifts I had to offer the world.

But to do that, I needed to embrace some things about myself, things I didn't even know brewed in my subconscious.

* * *

It's summer 2015. I'm on the mountainside, some hours out of cell range, with rolling hills of pine and aspens.

I'm with a group of 12 queer and trans people, and we're intention-setting before a rite of passage that involves four days of fasting.

Before me, a trans man with thick eyelashes and soft, buzzed hair crouches.

"Open the gates," he growls, low. Then louder, "Open the gates!"

Tears rip down his face, and a fire burns behind his eyes.

He raises his head to the sky and yells:

"Open the gates!"

His voice echoes off the mountains.

"Let me pass through," he quietly croaks.

I watch his chest rise and fall. I feel him at the crossroads, the threshold he needs to step through over which everything will change irrevocably.

Then, he stands and faces our guides to recite his intention:

"I am a gift from the divine feminine, and I'm whole through every part of my transition."

Our eyes lock, and something uncoils between us—a breath of *possible*.

* * *

The transgender, nonbinary, queer magic part of me needed a mirror so I could know how to name myself. I had known *of* a couple of transgender people in high school, but I didn't know their stories, and it never felt like an option available to me.

The only messages I heard about being trans were those stereotypical "I always knew," "I'm trapped in the wrong body" kinds of narratives. A cis-centric world wants to make *being transgender* the last option, an option only if your life is completely miserable without it. My life seemed pretty precarious, but I didn't think it was because I was trans.

In a community of queer people, witnessed by the ponderosa pine, I cut off all my hair to mark my transition into adulthood. Immediately afterward, I felt this stirring inside me, this tug to talk to the nonbinary people who were with me on that mountainside.

"What does the sacred masculine mean to you?" I found myself asking, and their answers began to unravel every gender box in my head.

Asking that question might have changed everything for me, because within 18 months, I started performing as a drag king, feeling like it was more a part of me than a costume. I joined a transgender choir, started using they/them pronouns, and took my first shot of testosterone. Something unnamed in me finally felt possible.

* * *

It's summer 2016.

Gender blossoms in every color within me, and I'm finally ready to show it.

I'm wearing shorts, with years-old self-harm scars still purple and raised from mapping my history on my legs. I don't cover them, but I don't feel thorns in them anymore. I hold my head high and slowly spin around the circle to meet the eyes of each queer person holding me as I speak:

"I am a soft, queer boy of infinite love. I'm a shapeshifter who knows wholeness on the changing wind. I am a guide who lusts for the voyage of the underworld."

My eyes land on Walker, a trans elder, age 50, inhabiting a wisdom old for his years but necessary for our community.

He takes my hands in his and says, "I see you, edgewalker. I see you, shapeshifter. I see that you need your underworld journeys—that's part of your gift. But you need to come back every time. Come back every time. Come back. Every. Time. Your community needs you to."

With those words, Walker gives me something my psychiatrist never could: a sense of belonging.

* * *

At last, I knew I had purpose. I knew I needed to commit to my lifeforce.

Finally, I realized after all my years of flirting with death, the most rewarding rebellion I could dance was that of self-love.

I try to find the words to explain the trauma of erasure. To explain the trauma of not having seen examples of myself—versions of myself happy and trans and alive.

When I look at my family tree, my hands trace the names of ancestors, cloaked in feminine and masculine labels, linked and remembered only by their heterosexuality. Floating over the branches, I linger in the absence, feeling all that's contained in our histories' silence. There's an unnamable grief within me when I reach for the faces of my queer heritage, wondering what stories and practices weren't passed down because of this erasure.

At the same time, there's something undeniably resilient about queer people. Though you can't trace us in your DNA, we've always been here. There has always been this thing that today, we call queerness. It's comforting and thrilling and humbling that no matter what I do, the future is filled with queer magic, and I get to be a part of it.

Today, I try to live into that creation, to let myself become again and again, to let myself be guided by queer joy, to express it so palpably that it sings permission to anyone who can really see me, to let loose a current of *possible* everywhere I walk.

Today, I write from constant bewilderment. I found it along a winding path, one that followed none of my haphazard maps. My legs still show the ways I've gone, but the truth of the matter is none of it could have been planned.

Even now, my time is not yet. I'm sure there will come a further day when grief will shatter my bones, when the demon whispers of self-destruction beckon me in turn, when the floods turn over and the forest burns down, but I will still be breathing.

When those times come, tears sleeting my eyes, I hope I bellow a resounding *thank you*. Because I will be alive, experiencing all the peculiar sorrows and joys that encompass a life, ever grateful that I get to *feel all of it*. Perhaps it's a blessed curse, but still, the richness of living courses through my veins. Even in my sorrow, I find it such a gift to experience life. That's the miracle of it all.

Instead of "remission," I get to experience my unique sense of joy. I find it dancing in my lovers' eyes, in the ghosts I talk to through piano strings, in the genderful voices of my beloved trans choir, in the resilience of the friends that come to candlelit vigils sobbing, and in this tantalizing belief that *the best things haven't happened yet.*

I know the worst things likely haven't happened yet either, but I'm convicted in seeing this world through.

Today, I stay alive for my queer and trans ancestors who couldn't. I stay alive for the young queer ones who may need to see that there's more possible in the world.

My elders made me promise to come back. I made a vow instead of a promise, since I was the type of cutter who always broke promises.

Trust me, I'll continue to walk the edges. They're terrifying and beautiful places to be, and I always taste like magic when I travel to them. But I vow to always come back.

I have to—

For you,

For my community,

For all of us,

and,

most importantly,

For me.

THE TOOL

SETUP

This is a trance to connect with your purpose. A trance is a state of enchantment, a way of sinking into the mythic landscape of your inner world, a way of listening to yourself.

Do whatever feels good for your body to deepen and surrender. You may want to sit, stand, or sway. You may want to dance. Perhaps you want to lie down.

Maybe you want to draw or write. Do whatever brings your senses most to life.

Perhaps you record yourself reading this back to yourself, or ask a friend to read it aloud. Perhaps you'll listen to my voice guide you at the link I've included at the end of this chapter.

TRANCE

Bring your awareness to your breath. Let your eyes go soft. Notice how deeply or shallowly you're breathing. Just notice. See if your breath changes just by bringing your awareness to it.

Bring your awareness to the darkness behind your eyelids. Let yourself sink into that dark. Submerge. Let the velvety dark wrap around you like a night sky folding over you or rich, dark soil. Keep submerging. Let your thoughts go quiet. Let the dark pull in your senses. Find yourself in a place of deep stillness.

From the stillness, let emerge a vast nighttime sky, an expanse of swirling cosmos. Maybe just one star twinkles at first—a blink, a wink glittering through the dark. Perhaps the galaxy, the vault of the Milky Way unfurls like currents across the curved edge of space. Marvel at the stars. See if the stars change just by bringing your awareness to them.

Marvel, and find in these stars a mirror. Marvel at the stars as if you are marveling at a mirror.

Find in this mirror your star—the star that is yours. Find in this mirror something of your essence. Something of your lifeforce. Something of your purpose. Imagine you can coax it towards you. Maybe you even say out loud: "Purpose, come to me." Draw it forth from this swirling galaxy. Draw it forth from this universe that contains *everything*, and also contains the essence of you. Call to your purpose.

What does your purpose feel like? Do the stars shift to make a constellation to show you? What does your purpose look like? What does your purpose sound like? How do you want to move when you reach for your purpose?

Notice everything, even the subtle. Embrace any flinch in your body, twitch in your toe.

Stare into the mirror of your purpose. Let it move you; let yourself imagine wildly.

Ask your purpose: "How do I honor you?"

Do this as long as it takes.

When you feel ready, call this purpose down. Let it fall from the great height of galaxies.

Call your purpose down.

Let it find the river of the Milky Way.

Let it swirl into the gravitational pull of Earth.

Let it course through layers of atmosphere.

Let it bathe in the light of the sun, reaching its rays around the planet.

Let it come down, down through the sky around you.

Let purpose land on your head. Let it twinkle like stars around the crown of your head. Maybe you even touch your skull. What does purpose feel like as it meets your skull?

Let it sink into your heart. What does purpose feel like here, in your heart?

Let your heart take this purpose and pump it through your veins. What does purpose feel like, as rivers that flow through you?

Let purpose fill you completely.

Breathe.

Notice your breath as you breathe with purpose.

Pat your body down.

Say your names out loud three times.

Look around your physical space and let yourself arrive fully back in the here and now.

A NOTE ON LINEAGE

I learned trance practice from the Reclaiming Witchcraft tradition, and this trance was inspired in part by the Star Goddess myth and my deep-self communing practice, from the triple soul framework of the Anderson Feri and Wildwood traditions. I honor these lineages that have given me so many tools, practices, and ways to become more fully myself in this world.

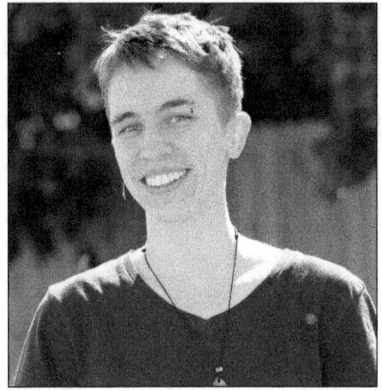

Silen Wellington (they/he) is a sculptor of sound, artist of people, storyteller, genderqueer shapeshifter, mercurial name collector, and lover, among other things. Avidly interdisciplinary, they make art as an act of service, healing, disruption, and magic, weaving together disciplines of poetry, acoustic sound, electronics, ritual, and performance art.

Silen is a white settler of primarily Norwegian and French descent living on Cheyenne, Arapaho, and Ute lands, seeking to unsettle himself and practice awareness and humility. Silen found their way to wholeness and self-love through mostly "alternative" means, namely: guided rites of passage journeys, performance art, unhinged-unfettered-unapologetic dance, and connections with fiercely humble elders and mentors who shared some of Silen's marginalized identities.

They have a BM in music composition and a BA in psychology from the University of Colorado Boulder. A wearer of many hats, Silen composes music, performs, writes, teaches witchcraft, provides peer support to those struggling with mental health, and offers spiritual coaching and mentorship.

In the world of peer support, Silen practices in the psychiatric survivor and Mad Pride lineages. They are a co-founder of a nonprofit in Northern Colorado called the Yarrow Collective, which offers anti-carceral mental health support alternatives that center consent, choice, and healing in community.

In the world of composing and music, Silen's work has been performed in gardens whispering delightful fae dances to the trans-ancestors that escape definition, featured boys in dresses next to saxophones, unveiled prescription label collages amid chaotic soundscapes of dysphoria, danced nonbinary shadow puppets behind sheets of rainbow light, and given permission to intramuscular testosterone injections under expansive life-giving harmonics.

In all aspects of their life, Silen aims to create spaces that provoke people to come closer to their authentic selves.

Connect with Silen:

Website: https://www.silenwellington.com

Instagram: https://www.instagram.com/silen_creature/

Trance Audio: https://silenwellington.com/purpose-trance

CHAPTER 10

One Choice Away: Break Free from Old Patterns

Tools for Personal Growth and Self-Love

Sue Bruckner, MA, LPC

I'm always just one choice away from loving myself better—and that truth defines my life.

This isn't just a nice saying for me; it's the thread that runs through my entire adult life, and the foundation of the work I now do every day.

I didn't arrive at this truth through ease. I arrived through heartbreak, pattern repetition, deep loss, and—if I'm completely honest—four men with beards, starting with my husband. Each relationship revealed something different about my wiring, my blind spots, and most importantly, my choices. Each bearded man represented a different pattern I needed to confront and heal—a mirror of the patterns I carried with me for years.

What started as a moment of clarity in my car became the foundation for everything I now teach other women—women who wake up one day and don't recognize the life they're living, who find themselves stuck in the same exhausting patterns in love, at work, and in the daily choices that somehow led them so far from who they're meant to be.

This is the story of how I learned to interrupt those patterns, one choice at a time.

And how you can, too.

MY STORY

My marriage unraveled, and I drowned in it.

Most mornings were some version of survival: two small kids melting down about going to school, a husband melting down about their meltdowns, and me, already exhausted before I reached my therapy practice, the only place that felt like a sanctuary.

I learned to take responsibility for my part in every conflict, searching for what I did wrong even when I couldn't see it. I apologized first, hoping he'd follow with ownership of his piece. He never did. Instead, he accepted my apology and told me I should have known better.

Whenever I tried to bring up something that hurt me, his response was always the same: "You make everything too hard." "I can never do anything right." "Why can't you just let things go?"

The pattern was always the same, no matter how gentle or careful I was.

That's when I discovered *Deal Breakers: When to Work on a Relationship and When to Walk Away,* by Dr. Bethany Marshall. On my daily drives, I listened to this audiobook—crying, laughing, sometimes screaming, and hitting the steering wheel. I rewound sections over and over, desperate for the validation this author gave me. Someone finally named what happened behind closed doors.

When I reached the section on partners who refuse to take responsibility, the author said it bluntly:

"You better get the highest dose of Prozac you can find."

The moment I heard those words, they landed in me like a full-body knowing.

No! I won't medicate myself to survive a marriage that requires me to disappear.

That moment in my car became one of the most defining moments of my life. It wasn't the first brave choice I'd made, but it was one of the clearest: the choice to believe I deserved better.

Not long after, I gifted myself a plaque that read: "She designed a life she loved." It became my daily permission slip—a quiet, steady reminder that I had agency. That I could choose differently. And so, I did.

Sometimes loving ourselves better is walking away from what we thought would be our forever.

* * *

As my marriage ended, I started dating again, beginning to learn what I really wanted in love. What I didn't realize was that each relationship—each bearded man—would teach me something different about my patterns and what I truly wanted.

The second bearded man came into my life when I desperately needed to feel wanted. His enthusiasm felt like oxygen after years of neglect. But over time, conversations always circled back to him, and I began to feel the familiar weight of someone else's stress and anxiety—a dynamic I left my marriage to escape. I also found myself longing for deep, honest conversations about growth and transformation—something entirely missing from both this relationship and my marriage.

I chose to believe a more aligned relationship was out there for me.

Then came the third bearded man—the one I brought to Colorado.

At first glance, he seemed like everything I had waited for: he meditated, practiced yoga, and spoke the language of personal growth. He said he wanted a woman who knew she was a goddess—strong, independent, grounded in her feminine. His words felt like an invitation to step fully into who I was.

But over time, I saw the gap between his words and his actions. His version of a goddess didn't allow space for my process or my voice when it differed from his. My love of growth and my attachment to potential made me susceptible to staying too long, convincing myself every conflict was just another opportunity to grow.

Before we left for Colorado—a three-week trip I knew would make or break the relationship—I told him it often felt like being on a leash: every time I expressed a thought or feeling he didn't like, he would yank. What I longed for was simple: "I'm so sorry. Let's figure this out." But that moment never came.

At a Colorado campground with my closest friends, I rounded the corner and saw him.

He was dominating the conversation, talking over them, seemingly unaware of his impact. I stopped walking. Something shifted in my chest as I watched this scene unfold: my people, who knew me so well, were being steamrolled —a dynamic I knew all too well.

The pattern crystallized with brutal clarity: men who talk more than they listen, who take space but don't hold space. The recognition hit like a physical force.

Later, one of my friends gently observed, "You like the talkers."

"Yes," I replied dryly, still processing what I witnessed. "I have a pattern."

During that trip, *Untamed* by Glennon Doyle traveled with me. Her two questions became my compass: "Is it true? Is it beautiful?" The answers came quickly, each time I was interrupted or dismissed: *No. No. No.*

I also carried a question adapted from Kamal Ravikant's work that I teach my clients: "If I loved myself fully and truly, would I allow this moment?" The answer was equally clear.

By the time we returned from Colorado, I knew. I ended the relationship with certainty, boundaries, and righteous self-love. No more explaining, no more managing his anger, no more convincing.

The pattern interrupting didn't stop there; it continued.

* * *

After years of gradually interrupting my patterns, I continued making different choices. Three months later, I met the fourth bearded man—someone who listened and held space. Yet, I struggled with receiving what I always craved.

"I eat kindness." These words tumbled out of my mouth in the early days with my now-partner, my kind-hearted, bearded love. What I meant surprised me: I consume kindness but struggle to take it in. When it comes from romantic partners, I push back and question its authenticity, often meeting it with sarcasm.

Standing in the unfamiliar space of being loved well, I was struck by how foreign it felt.

When kindness came from men, my nervous system braced. I tightened. Part of me questioned if it was real. Part of me assumed it meant something must be lacking in him—that loving me so freely had to signal weakness.

I spent so much of my life knocking—on doors, on hearts—trying to be seen in many of my significant relationships: 12 years with a partner who couldn't see me, and family relationships where I longed for attention and curiosity about my life. I was the one reaching, asking to be loved more fully. And when love was finally offered without effort—without earning—it felt disorienting. My system didn't know how to receive it.

I chose to stay curious about my internal words and feelings that accompanied his kindness, and they kept leading me to the same judgment: that he lacked self-esteem. I kept hearing, *He's only kind to you because he's weak.* But I didn't embrace this as truth—I knew it was something about my own beliefs. It was clear I had work to do.

I used a technique from my training to investigate what drove this resistance. The belief I uncovered made me gasp: *To love me fully is a weakness.*

That realization stopped me; it wasn't truth, just a survival story—a belief I created based on a lifetime of working to be seen. If I had to wave for 12 years to get my partner's attention, if I had to create openings for family members to be curious about my life, then surely anyone who saw me easily and loved me freely must be missing something. It was easier to question their depth than to believe I deserved effortless love.

A pattern. And like every pattern I interrupted before, I chose to meet it with curiosity, not judgment.

My truth is: I'm worthy of kindness, generosity, and love. My truth is: Love doesn't have to be earned through struggle.

This relationship became the safest place I've ever done my work. After years of navigating dysregulated partners, raising children alone, and running a household and a business—often carrying everything myself—I'm learning to soften. To lean into shared leadership. To receive.

He remembers details from conversations weeks ago and asks follow-up questions about my work, feelings, and dreams—not because he has to, but because he's genuinely curious about my inner world. Sometimes I catch myself thinking, *Is this what emotional intimacy with a man looks like?* The deep conversations, the genuine interest in who I am beyond what I can give him—this is what I always craved but never experienced with a romantic partner.

My stomach's clenching is the first clue I receive his kindness as people-pleasing, one of his tendencies he's actively working to shift. I'm so acutely aware of how my body responds; it's my truth barometer. I share with him my experience of his kindness, and he'll take a vulnerable look inward to see what his motivation was. Was it people-pleasing, or was it his love for his goddess? I can't say I'm always right, and I value being humbled. It's a dance, and a clumsy one at times, but over our years together, we're finding our rhythm. He knows I don't want cheerleading, but that I do want to be seen.

And that's what we both bring: ownership and humility. He does his work. He takes responsibility for his part without defensiveness. Being with someone who owns his piece has been eye-opening; I see how easy it would be to let him carry it all, the way others once let me. That insight has made me even more committed to owning mine.

His accountability highlighted what was missing all along.

He's redefining manhood with great commitment to doing the hard internal work. Sensitive, deep, caring—without apology. He actively chooses what masculinity means to him, embracing emotional availability and deep listening despite cultural pressure that tells him these qualities make him less of a man. He's wildly brave in his vulnerability, something

I never witnessed in a partner. He rejects toxic masculinity and takes pride in building something new.

A big part of my work now is this ongoing discernment: Is this my authentic self responding or my conditioned self? It's the question that keeps me growing, keeps me choosing love over fear.

* * *

These weren't just relationships. They were my training ground.

As I loved myself better, one beard at a time, I started noticing patterns not just in my partners, but in myself: my tolerance for being unseen, my attachment to potential, my fear of receiving kindness, my belief that struggle was necessary for growth.

And as I became more curious—rather than judgmental—about those patterns, a set of tools began to emerge. I learned them while standing in the middle of my patterns, adapting wisdom from various sources, asking better questions, and making different choices, one vulnerable moment at a time. Over years of loving myself better, I've distilled what works into simple but profound practices that help my clients interrupt the same exhausting patterns that once kept me stuck.

I want to share those tools with you here because you, too, are always one choice away.

THE TOOL

YOUR ONE CHOICE AWAY METHODOLOGY STARTER KIT

We aren't broken; we're simply conditioned. And when we meet that conditioning with curiosity instead of judgment, everything shifts.

These three tools are your starter kit: the essential practices I teach every client to begin interrupting patterns and choosing themselves differently. While there are deeper layers to explore, these foundational tools will give you everything you need to start loving yourself better today.

1. POWER QUESTIONS: YOUR INTERNAL COMPASS

What it is: Three specific questions that cut through emotional overwhelm and create instant clarity in difficult moments.

When to use it:

- When you're unsure whether to stay or go in any situation.
- During conflict, uncomfortable conversations, or when second-guessing your instincts.
- Before making any decision that feels heavy.

The three questions:

"Is it true? Is it beautiful?"

- Use this when someone is speaking to you or about you.
- Trust your body's immediate response.
- If the answer is no to either question, you have information.

"If I loved myself fully, would I allow this moment?"

- Use this to cut through wishful thinking, potential, and old conditioning.
- Forces you to stand in what's happening, not what you wish might happen.
- Brings you back to self-honoring in real-time.

"Is this a life I love?"

- Use this as a daily check-in, especially during transitions.
- If the answer is no, follow up with: "What one choice would move me closer?"

Practice this: Choose one of these questions to use for the next week. Notice what insights arise and how your decision-making shifts when you have a clear internal compass.

2. HOW I WANT TO FEEL: YOUR EMOTIONAL GPS

What it is: A practice of choosing your emotional state first, then taking actions that support that feeling, rather than trying to control external circumstances to feel better.

When to use it:

- Before challenging conversations or anxiety-provoking events.
- When you notice yourself trying to control others' behavior.
- During times of uncertainty or transition.

How to use it:

1. Name two ways you want to feel (confident, calm, grounded, peaceful).
2. Identify two to three small actions within your control that support these feelings.
3. Take action on these before the situation occurs.

Examples:

- Want to feel confident before a difficult conversation? Wear clothes that make you feel strong, practice what you want to say, and do breathwork.
- Want to feel peaceful during family conflict? Set a boundary about topics you won't discuss, bring headphones, and have an exit strategy.

Practice this: Before your next challenging situation, ask: "How do I want to feel?" Then identify three specific actions you can take to support that feeling. Notice how this shifts your experience.

3. I AM, YOU ARE: YOUR CENTERING TECHNIQUE

What it is: A simple phrase that creates space between who you are and what's happening around or within you, preventing you from absorbing others' emotions or being hijacked by your own reactions.

When to use it:

- When someone comes home in a bad mood, you feel yourself tensing.
- When anxiety, shame, or old fears surface.
- During emotionally charged conversations.
- When you notice yourself taking on others' energy.

How to use it:

1. Identify what you're witnessing (an emotion, behavior, or energy).

2. Separate yourself using this phrase: "I am [your name]. You are [the thing you're witnessing]."

3. Breathe and notice the space this creates.

Examples:

- "I am Sarah. You are my partner's frustration."

- "I am Sarah. You are anxious about tomorrow."

- "I am Sarah. You are a conditioned thought that no longer serves me."

Practice this: Use this technique three times this week—once with someone else's emotion, once with your own emotion, and once with a limiting belief. Notice how it feels to witness rather than absorb.

* * *

Four beards. Four relationships. Four invitations to love myself better.

What started as a pattern of attraction became a path of deep transformation—from someone who believed love required struggle to a woman who finally allows herself to receive kindness. The most profound shift? Realizing that joy has as much to teach us as pain does.

Sometimes loving ourselves better means walking away from what we once hoped would last. Sometimes it means interrupting a pattern with compassion instead of shame. Sometimes it means finally accepting the very kindness we've always craved.

You, too, are always just one choice away from loving yourself better. The tools I've shared are your first step toward that freedom.

Your one-choice-away moment is waiting. What will you choose?

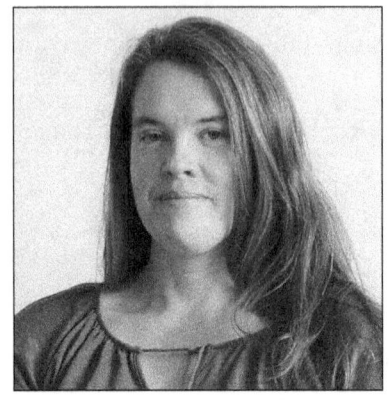

Sue Bruckner, MA, LPC, is a holistic relationship coach, licensed professional counselor, and founder of With Intention and Tribe Rising. Sue helps women who feel everything deeply, overthink every decision, and have been people-pleasing for so long they've forgotten what they actually want.

Drawing from over a decade of psychotherapy practice and her own lived journey through divorce and rebuilding, Sue guides these women through life's most complex transitions with calm and clarity. Her work is built on the truth that sustainable growth only comes from love, not fear—a lesson learned through her pattern of relationships that taught her how to interrupt cycles and choose herself.

At the heart of Sue's methodology is the One Choice Away framework, a blend of nervous system regulation, spiritual alignment, and practical tools that helps women break exhausting patterns and cultivate deep emotional safety, particularly with themselves.

Sue's approach blends her psychotherapy background with somatic regulation and mindset tools, teaching women to trust their inner wisdom and navigate overwhelming emotions with grace. She believes sensitive women don't need fixing—they need witnessing, regulation, support, and permission to honor their emotional truth.

Through her Tribe Rising membership community, private coaching, and group programs, Sue creates sacred spaces where women can heal not in isolation, but in connection with others who truly understand. Her work emphasizes that being witnessed by emotionally safe people accelerates healing and reduces the chaos of rebuilding.

When she's not coaching, Sue can be found with her two children and kindhearted, bearded partner, caring for their menagerie of pets at home or escaping to their cabin in the woods with their dog, the freckled menace—living proof that patterns can be interrupted, and joy can become our teacher.

Connect with Sue:

Website: http://www.suebruckner.com/

Email: suebruckner@withintentioncoaching.com

Free One Sentence Truth Guide: https://bit.ly/onesentencetruthHCH

CHAPTER 11

Thank You Divorce

Expectant Gratitude After Heartbreak

Madisen Rose

MY STORY

"I should have divorced you so much sooner."

We're sitting on the curb in front of the duplex he's moving into. I didn't know anything about his new place until I saw the bed of his yellow truck full of furniture on my usual route home from work.

I still live in the house we rented as newlyweds. We're eight months into the separation and my nonprofit salary can't keep up.

The hope that he'd move home—and the monthly $500 float from my dad to ensure my rent check cleared—are what kept me in our place.

This was how things were the last two years. He made decisions. I stepped on landmines. Landmines like the furniture in the truck bed belonging to his new roommate—oh, wait, his girlfriend.

On our wedding day, I vowed, "With the love in my heart and the power of God to help me, I vow to stand by your side, to journey with you, to care for you, respect you, protect you, edify and serve you with all that I have. I vow to be your confidante and your most dedicated companion."

Maybe I took the "most dedicated companion" part a little too far. I held on, believing we could restore the marriage, that we could start over, that we could repair with "God on our side."

I gave myself fully to this man-my devotion, my hope, and my silence. I continued to expose my tender underbelly as the young wife who would never speak ill of her husband. I was willing to sacrifice anything, even myself. I thought, *if only he could see my heart, he would choose me again and move back home.*

Divorce did things to my faith. It gave me something to cling to in the chaos and confusion. The community of people who said, "I'll pray for you," gave me comfort. Getting divorced challenged how I thought I was supposed to live and expanded the edges of my concept of spirituality. I tried desperately to follow the traditional path, and when my marriage broke, so did my view of the world, and the supposed benefit of obedience.

We "did everything right." I couldn't accept that the marriage was over. Even the day we met with the judge to submit the final paperwork, we waited in the hall at the courthouse, and I offered, "We don't have to do this."

"We do," he said.

We sat on another curb that day, and I'm glad I had tissues with me because we both needed them. "I'll always love you," pinged my soul tie.

They say, "When you know, you know," when finding "the one."

I knew, which is why I vowed to give him all I had. I did. I never thought I'd believe this, but I'm grateful to my ex-husband for doing the thing I couldn't do.

I would've stayed.

We were the couple with the big yard that hosted everyone's birthday celebrations and going-away parties. Behind closed doors, I didn't know how to reveal myself. I thought being low maintenance was the key to sustaining a marriage, but it's interpreted as apathy. Internally, I was a swirl of desperate loneliness and stinging rage because I had lost control. Manipulation is not the path to connection. I know that now.

We prioritized maintaining the façade because we couldn't risk judgment, losing credibility, or, God forbid, having anyone think less of us for struggling to know ourselves and each other. The first year of marriage is supposed to be the hardest, but for us, it was year two. "You'll figure it out," they say, but no one talked to us about what happens when you can't.

I tried to convince myself we were just going through a rough patch, right? Glimpses of reconciliation kept me going, like renewing our lease before hosting our annual Saint Patrick's Day party, even though no one knew he'd been staying somewhere else for three months.

Our little house smelled like cabbage for days after the party where our friends gathered around two tables pushed together. But they weren't the same height, so there was no sliding to pass the potatoes. Three people were on the couch like a bench, but they sat awkwardly low with the squish of the cushions, so that's where the tall guests went.

We had everything: dark beer, corned beef, Irish soda bread, butter, and mustard.

Everything looks perfect. Then, *pffffthhhhppppptttt.*

A hair.

GRATITUDE AS A GATEWAY TO TRUST

I don't remember where the suggestion of gratitude came from. It could've been one of the five bullet points from my internet search of "getting through divorce" or the inspirational agenda item at my work retreat.

I would try anything, so I started a daily gratitude practice. Here's the unedited list, a mere thirteen days into separation.

January 9, 2017

1. I am thankful for the coffee and cherries in my smoothie

2. I am grateful for friends and birthdays. Happy B-day Tasha!

3. Encouraging friends who speak life over me

4. Bible study ladies as sister prayer warriors

5. Resources available on the internet

6. Technology and access to so many great books/articles, etc.

7. Self-talk and Shad Helmstetter

8. Loving, praying parents

9. Cute shoes

10. A healthy body and great hair!

Starting somewhere small, like the people around me, what I ate, or access to information, was all I had energy for. This was where I had to begin with gratitude to try to introduce something other than the list of 100 things that made it hard to breathe.

The gratitude practice became my buoy during the most heartbreaking years of my life. The first thing I did when I sat down at my desk in the morning was try to think of a few good things. It became a way for me to ground when, *this is not my life,* was on replay.

It was like I looked at my life in one of those distorted mirrors in a carnival funhouse for two years. After a while, when it's all you can see, you start to believe it.

The gratitude practice was like the tiny mirror in the lid of a compact. It's small, so you can only see it up close, like your upper lip or one eye. Gratitude anchored me in a new reality until I was confident enough in my own perception to believe what I saw in the full-length mirror.

Perspective is everything.

HOUSE LIGHTS UP

I stood on a stage. The spotlight was blinding, so all I could really see was the circle of light a few feet around me. A fresh candy apple red pedi prepped me for the summer, and I held a paper to-go cup of coffee.

If I squinted, I could see someone sitting on the ground in the shadows. She wasn't looking at me, but I could tell she was there.

It seemed like I stood there in silence for an eternity. I kept looking at the ground and down at myself, my brass key ring tucked into the small front pocket of my black skinny jeans. My stomach growled. All I could see was what was in the spotlight. Everything else was so dark.

What's going on?

Where is everyone?

"Hello? Can someone turn on the house lights?"

As the lights faded on, I made out the audience's faces. Every seat was filled with someone who loved me in some way. My family, my friends, my barista, my clients, my coworkers, my friends' kids, my neighbor, my landlord. All these witnesses were there the entire time.

I could also see scenes from my dreams, the future, beach days, my home, and everything I've ever wanted.

Gratitude in the midst of heartbreak is like only being able to see what's in the spotlight. We know there's more than what we can see in the little ring of light. We can't see in the dark, so we need to bring the house lights up. That's what abundance reminds us of. There's so much there, we have to have the eyes and the light to see it.

I got *really* good at gratitude. I held both things: my grief and my gratitude.

There were more and more mornings I woke up without puffy eyes or a pile of used tissues on the floor next to the bed. Wincing in the produce section became less frequent. Red bell peppers were always on the list, but they weren't for me. I never had to buy them again.

The basics consumed my days. Drink water. Remember to eat something. Try to breathe, but not too deeply, because then I would cough or cry, and I was so tired of crying.

The house stayed virtually the same from the time he moved out until we broke the lease, except for the ridiculous amount of plants I got for free on Facebook Marketplace. I had to have something to take care of other than myself because confronting all the ways I had abandoned myself in the midst of the divorce was too much.

Shortly after the conversation on the curb about the furniture in the yellow truck bed, I found somewhere else to live that I could afford.

It was a basement.

It was always a basement.

Packing up the cabinets filled with items from the wedding gift registry transitioned to observing quiet hours and reminders about which knife didn't go in the dishwasher. I put my life in painful boxes and stuffed myself into the extra bedroom for out-of-town guests.

I lived in the "lower level" for two years at one address and nine months at another. When I told myself, *No more basements,* I knew something was shifting. I believed I could ask for more than what the older couple at church who wanted to help me out generously offered. Don't get me wrong. I was so grateful to have a place to live that fit my budget, but I wanted more.

I wanted up and out.

Thankfully, I was able to do both—get out of the basements and into a place above ground—a second-story studio corner unit with windows on three sides. This was the first place where I had a fridge all to myself. Dreamy. Adding ten things to my gratitude list each day was easy that month.

Hey reader, now that you've read about the power of gratitude in the midst of my heartbreak, we're going to shift gears a bit. We're going to start with straightforward gratitude for what is and move beyond that to an expectant gratitude practice called Abundance Flows.

THE TOOL

A typical gratitude practice lists what's already present in your life. You might be grateful for the sunshine, for coffee, or for the people who mean the most to you.

Gratitude is not toxic positivity. There's no denying that there will be days that feel unbearable. We're not only looking at the good and ignoring the bad.

This tool consists of two parts. We'll start with a basic gratitude practice framework and take it to the next level with an expectant gratitude practice called Abundance Flows.

If you're reading this, I'd guess you've gone through some things. You might be thinking, "Gratitude. Really? You can't be serious. My life is imploding. What could I possibly be grateful for?"

Stay with me on this one. I've rolled my eyes at cliches like "You find what you look for," but it turns out to be science.

If you truly practice gratitude, it's life-changing because it has been shown to reduce blood pressure and regulate breathing to synchronize with the heartbeat.

Gratitude physiologically changes the neural structures in your brain, according to the UCLA Mindfulness Awareness Research Center.

Gratitude changed my neuropathways. By practicing gratitude, you create patterns in your brain, so you'll be able to scan and recognize when something registers as an addition to your list.

When you experience a low period, loss, major change, or especially significant life transitions, giving yourself something to consider beyond heartache stretches the edges of your focus (think spotlight) and gives you a little margin.

Margin for a deeper breath.

Margin for a smile.

Margin for a laugh.

Margin for a welcome distraction.

TOOL PART 1: GRATITUDE PRACTICE

Let's get practical first:

1. Where: Decide where you'll document your gratitude.

   - Handwritten on a calendar, in a journal, or digitally, like the notes app on your phone.

   - Be realistic about what you will *actually* do.

2. When: Pick a time when you'll make your list consistently.

   - Make it easy on yourself and incorporate your gratitude practice into your existing routine, so it feels less like one more thing on your plate.

   - Let it be the first thing you do when you sit down at your desk for work or while you wait for the coffee to brew.

   - Keep a running list with dates.

3. 10: List ten things each day that you're grateful for.

- Big
- Small
- The same as yesterday
- No self-judgment or shame
- They don't have to make sense to anyone else
- Be as consistent as possible

There might be days when coming up with a list of ten seems impossible. This is why it's essential to write it down. You don't need to rely on your recall, and feel free to copy and paste from the day before if needed.

Some mornings, what made my list was as simple as my car starting, health insurance, or a good hair day, probably because I washed it after wearing it in a messy bun for four days.

Other times, what made the list was a little bit deeper. Here are a few excerpts from the lists in 2017:

- hard conversations
- a little bit of anger
- knowing I did everything I could think of
- knowing that some things are hard, but it doesn't make them bad
- no next step has to be forced; there is no timeline, only what feels right to me
- new sense of home
- being able to apologize
- realizing I'm not perfect and I never will be, but I can still be used and have a vision for my life
- understanding my value

TOOL PART 2: ABUNDANCE FLOWS

After consistently practicing gratitude during my years of separation, divorce, and beyond, I became accustomed to paying attention to what was present. After stabilizing, I could pay attention to more.

I started noticing the extras, the bonuses, the discounts, gifts, and the overflow. I began to call it abundance because it was so much more than what I needed. It's the extra special, unexpected, or a surprise I didn't see coming, or have the awareness to ask for.

Abundance Flows is an expectant take on a typical gratitude practice. You may not know what delights are in store, but you believe they're coming. You are expecting abundance to make its way to you without knowing how.

Whatever method you decide to use for your gratitude practice, do the same thing for your Abundance Flows practice.

Where: Decide on a location where you'll document.

When: Pick a time.

Add dates to the list as things arise.

You may not have ten things each day, but you might! Here are a few examples from my Abundance Flows list:

- Berries were on sale two for one
- I won concert tickets at that free networking event
- Front row parking when I was running late today
- The server let us keep the mozzarella sticks sent to our table by mistake
- Free community yoga
- The box of crystals and stones from Heather before her move to Italy
- Freshly baked cookies from a friend
- I got to carpool to Denver
- Free shipping and a holiday discount

Once you start seeing the overflow, you'll continue to see Abundance Flows. These gifts will continue to show up. This is why we practice Abundance Flows—not just to notice, but to expect.

Consider this: the things you're adding to your Abundance Flows list have been present all along. Maybe you couldn't recognize them before because it's dark on the days that feel like survival.

Get the house lights up. Abundance Flows.

And no matter what, dear reader, consider me a friend, a guide, a mirror. I'm available to support you, a loved one, or a child in the unique and complex aftermath of divorce you might find yourself in.

Gratitude will ground you.

Abundance Flows will expand you.

Today, I'm adding you to my gratitude list.

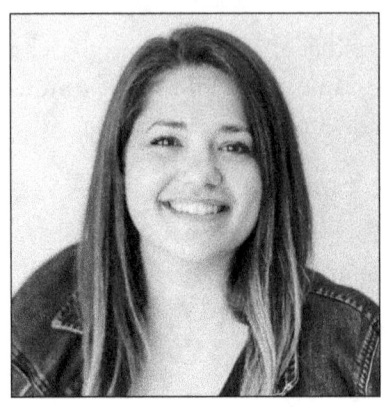

Madisen Rose is the founder and CEO of Better Half to Whole, a platform dedicated to supporting individuals through divorce recovery and the renegotiation of relational trauma in the nervous system. Through digital resources, self-paced online courses, group programs, and one-on-one sessions, Madisen helps people rebuild after divorce with intention, grit, and self-trust. These practical resources focus on the social and emotional aspects of life after divorce, like how to respond to "How are you?" and navigating shifts in family dynamics and the day-to-day.

A fourth-generation Colorado-born, Madisen brings a diverse background in hospitality, customer service, international sales, nonprofit fundraising, and 13 years of wedding coordination and event planning to her work. Her deep belief in the power of human connection and creative expression continues to shape her work today.

When she's not posting her cappuccinos on Instagram, you can find her on a paddleboard, planning her next international trip, practicing Spanish, or in a deep conversation about the quiet parts of ourselves that come out to play when it's safe.

Madisen's own healing pursuits include everything from somatic experiencing, talk therapy, acupuncture, and EMDR to singing bowl meditations and spirit baths. Now a somatic practitioner, she specializes in helping clients gently renegotiate relational trauma through embodied, trauma-trained practices, supporting the entire family after divorce, including the children, through nervous system work. Madisen is passionate about building community, supporting women, children, and families, and bridging the space between science and the sacred.

For a downloadable PDF of the Abundance Flows tool, go to www.betterhalftowhole.com/healingcurious.

Because everyone deserves access to information, especially in the early days after divorce, Madisen created the free online mini-course

Divorced. Now What? designed to guide you from "I don't know how I'm going to get through this" to "I'm ready to begin again."

In the mini-course, you'll learn concepts like how to get support when you don't know what you need, taking things one day at a time by going back to the basics, and navigating alone time, overwhelm, and decision fatigue.

By the end of the mini-course, you'll feel steadier, moving forward — one real day at a time with support, reclaiming a sense of control through small, meaningful decisions, and start to welcome new experiences that feel like you again.

Access the mini-course **Divorced. Now What?** here: https://better-half-to-whole.teachable.com/p/divorced-now-what

Connect with Madisen:

Website: www.betterhalftowhole.com

Email: madisen@betterhalftowhole.com

Instagram: https://www.instagram.com/betterhalftowhole/

Facebook: https://tinyurl.com/BHTWFacebook

LinkedIn: www.linkedin.com/in/madisen-rose-50b9691a

CHAPTER 12

Unmuted

Reclaim Your Voice Through Music and Memory

Lisa Boate

MY STORY

I am on the other side of everything I ever imagined for my life.

And for the first time, I realized—I never once considered what comes next.

That thought became the catalyst for my midlife revolution. It all began on an early spring morning, the kind that makes you believe in fresh starts. I sat on my deck, wrapped in the quiet comfort of a warm cup of tea, the sun on my face, the world around me bursting into a thousand shades of green. For a moment, I felt a rare sense of peace—like maybe I had done everything right.

And then that peace became eerily silent as a note of discord began to emanate from the depths of my heart.

I was absorbing the life I had built—one that, from the outside, looked exactly as it should. I followed the choreography laid out for women like me: coming of age in the late '80s and early '90s, our lives shaped by John Hughes movies, montages of struggle to success set to epic power ballads, and scripts about who we should be. We were taught how to perform our way through girlhood, motherhood, and career-building.

And I did. I built a meaningful career in education. I partnered with a man I love deeply. We poured ourselves into raising two phenomenal young humans. I had checked every box.

But when the steps in the dance ran out, I was left standing still, wondering:

How did I get here?

Who am I now?

And what do I actually want?

In the creation of a life, in all the doing, I lost my being.

As my intentionally crafted roles evolved, I quite suddenly had more time because my boys didn't need me in the same immediate ways. The daily rhythm of motherhood changed. My career, once a source of pride, now triggered so much anxiety that I cried on the way to work and lost clumps of hair from stress. I noticed that the once sure and steady choreography felt like chaos and frenzy.

Along with the tears and the hair evacuating my head, there were thousands of messages from my body that something wasn't right. I stumbled over the choreographed steps for years, but I just kept hurtling myself through space, telling my body to behave, to be quiet, to follow the fucking directions.

In a moment, the music of my heart, mind, soul, and body began to wildly shift in tempo, so I couldn't continue to fake my way through steps that no longer felt good in my body. It was time to listen and lean into the shifting tempo rather than resist it.

In letting go of the resistance, I made space for a realization. It was time to reclaim the music my soul loved to dance to and freestyle the movement because my body needed to break free of the prescribed steps that kept me small.

That's when the walls I created to form the facade of my identity begin to crumble.

I started asking, "Who am I without the roles? Without the titles?"

Mother, teacher, daughter, caregiver—those are *roles*. But society told me that's who I am. So, when those roles began to shift and disappear, it shook the foundation of my identity.

Yes, I will always be a mother. But not in the same way. The urgency of their needs is gone. The job description has changed. And I hadn't prepared for what that meant—for how deeply it would impact my sense of self.

So I got up with that cup of tea and went back into the house.

Jolted.

And thought: *Now what?*

I spent years creating a life that supported everyone else. But was it *my* life? Was *I* truly reflected in it? I wasn't sure.

That morning, something cracked open in me. It was the beginning of a shift that's still unfolding—a journey that is unfamiliar, uncomfortable, liberating, and terrifying all at once.

Because getting to know myself again means confronting truths. It means reckoning with the infrastructure I built around who I was *expected* to be.

I was taught to be busy. It's the currency of success in our culture: kids in activities, careers in overdrive, house curated, meals perfected— because being busy keeps us from asking the dangerous questions.

What do I really want?

Am I truly happy?

Who am I, really?

When I finally slowed down enough to ask the hard questions, I stepped into something powerful. I became a woman who started challenging the lyrics, and that was unsettling. For the systems around me, yes—but also terrifying for me.

Asking those questions is what ultimately brought me to the end of my teaching career.

Because when I finally asked myself, *Who am I?* and *What do I want?* "Teacher" was not the answer.

From my very earliest experience with the education system, the universe whispered: *This place isn't for you.*

Before I ever stepped into a classroom, I was full of music and magic. Curious, creative, mischievous—I asked questions, shared what I thought, and absorbed the beautiful music of the world around me. I was always learning, just not in traditional ways.

In kindergarten, I remember the windows. A giant bank of them stretched across one wall, and I sat there, staring out at the dancing trees, aching to be *out there*—in the vastness, the freedom—not stuck in this constricting box.

It took no time for me to get the message: *You are too much for this place.*

I sat next to my best friend. We created joyful noise together, giggling and sharing secrets, so the teacher moved me to a table of boys, thinking those boys would teach me my place, quiet and small. It didn't work.

That same afternoon, I came to school brimming with excitement, bursting to share what I learned that morning. I watched Canada AM with my mom, and there was a segment on Galapagos turtles that ignited my five-year-old imagination. I arrived at school and couldn't wait to share what I learned with the boys at my table.

That's when my teacher snapped. Furious, she stormed over, angry that I—seated where I was supposed to be tamed—led the conversation. She moved me again. This time to a desk at the front of the room. Alone. Facing the wall.

I remember that moment with piercing clarity.

That little girl knew.

This place was not made for her.

And yet, a mechanism inside me clicked.

I'll earn their approval.

So I became small. Quiet. Compliant. I quieted the original music I created, and I stepped into the 'good girl' choreography. I followed that choreography with painstaking precision. I got the grades. I was praised—a role model for how well I played small. I was celebrated for how well I learned to mute myself.

That message never changed even as I moved through my career.

Be quiet, be small, don't ask questions. As long as you continue not to stand out in this choir of conformity, you'll belong here.

The moment I began stepping into my real voice—as a woman, as a leader—the system pushed back. Hard.

After several years as a central resource teacher, our workspace was being reorganized. I went to move my things in, and the principal stopped me.

"That desk isn't for you. You're over here."

"Over here" was a desk, in the corner, as disconnected from the rest of the team as possible. I turned and looked at the spaces, and something deep in my subconscious let go. A towering wave of grief rose up, and I had to make a very quick exit to the washroom where I let the wave overtake me. I sobbed, body wracking wails that seriously alarmed the woman in the stall next to me.

I didn't understand why I was so gutted until I realized I was continuing to live the same story. I was being put in the corner. Again.

And it didn't stop.

As the year went on, I was shuffled deeper and deeper into the margins until finally, I worked in a literal closet, under a staircase.

The universe brought me full circle, to my kindergarten self.

Separated. Controlled. My curiosity, my passion, my impishness tucked away where they couldn't influence anyone else. Again, I was muted; people with power rejected my song. The worst part was that I could no longer hear myself. In every instance of resistance, I let the system change me. I let it mute my song until there was only silence, but this time, instead of blending into the orchestra that actively rejected me, I let my original score flow freely.

I decided I mattered. I decided I was no longer willing to contort myself to fit inside an institution that wouldn't hear me. In the end, I surrendered-not because I was lost—but because I realized:

I was meant to be music, melodic and free, I was put on this Earth to use my voice and to amplify others, not to perpetuate the quiet of conformity.

So I resigned, because staying would've cost me everything. It was time to reach back to that brave, curious, powerful little girl and say:

"I didn't forget you. I'm choosing you now. It's time to reclaim our beautiful music."

That music had been silent for a very long time. As I tentatively choreographed my next step, I knew that to pump up my own volume, there would need to be joy, fun, and a whole lot of magic.

One day, many months later, I pulled a fragrant, fresh loaf of bread out of the oven and rocked out to a solo dance party in my kitchen. My youngest son walked in and said, "Oh, there you are."

I often wonder how long he searched for me, to see the me he knew before I was turned all the way off. That moment was the clearest sign that I was coming back to life—my volume rising, my voice no longer on mute.

It was the first note on a brand new soundtrack I finally curated for myself.

THE TOOL

As you read my story, I hope you picked up on the musical theme. This theme has been preparing you for the fun and creative tool I have created to help you reconnect to yourself, time-traveling through music to remember who you were, so you can dream forward about who you are becoming.

Throughout my life, I have always found music to be the place I go to feel.

It is a deeply sensory modality that connects us with all our senses. When I hear a song that has powerful resonance for me, of course, I listen to it and feel the vibration of the music in my body. I also feel the warm breezes on my skin, smell the freshness of lake-infused air at dusk, feel my feet dancing in unison with the people I love, or taste salty tears on my tongue as a song releases a wave of grief. In the wise words of Amy Camie, Therapeutic Clinical Musician:

"Music can be a profound step in the exploration of self, in the conscious act of honest reflection that goes by many names–mindfulness, meditation, self-discovery, self-empowerment, and enlightenment."

Music is the most profound way I've experienced to consciously reflect on my lived experiences and how those experiences play together in the woman I am right now. Music is the one thing that cuts through all my numbness. It melts the ice I have spent a life building up around all my soft spots-my body's attempt to keep me safe and steady. I know now the numbness kept me distant from pain, fear, and grief; it also kept me from feeling joy, wonder, and excitement.

Creating my personal soundtrack has been the most beautiful way to open up my heart to feel in ways that allow me to heal.

If you'd like some inspiration, check out my podcast episode where I dance you through my soundtrack, Transforming 45: "The Soundtrack of my life in 15 Songs," and the process I used to create it. The link is available at the end of this chapter.

I hope you find joy in this creative process. Let yourself go, get lost in the depths of your sensory memory; your soundtrack is waiting to be heard.

THE SOUNDTRACK OF YOU: A TOOL FOR RECLAIMING VOICE AND MEMORY

Your life has a soundtrack. Not just a collection of favorite songs, but a curated playlist of the moments that shaped you—the joy, the grief, the awakenings, and the transformations.

This tool, The Soundtrack of You, is a process I created that bridges memory, emotion, and somatic reconnection. It's playful and surprisingly healing. Below, I'll walk you through how to build your own life soundtrack and use it as a doorway back to yourself.

STEP 1: SET YOUR INTENTION

Begin by deciding on a loose structure. I started by asking myself: *What are the 10 songs that define me?* I quickly realized that ten wasn't enough, so I expanded to 15. You might need more or fewer. This isn't about rules; it's about resonance. Let 15 be a soft limit that keeps the process doable while allowing space for complexity.

Tip: This is not a "greatest hits" playlist. This is a memory soundtrack. Let the songs choose you.

STEP 2: LET THE SONGS COME TO YOU

Don't overthink it. Sit down, take a few deep breaths, and let the songs surface. Ask yourself:

- What songs have never left me?
- What music played during key turning points in my life?
- What do I hear that makes my body remember something before my mind does?

Make a messy list. Don't worry about chronology yet, let the music rise from the depths.

STEP 3: SIT WITH EACH SONG

Give each song your full attention. Put on your headphones. Don't multitask. Just *listen*.

Then, ask:

- What emotions arise in my body?
- What do I see, smell, taste, or touch when I hear this?
- Who was I when I first heard it? Who am I now?
- Why did this song choose me?

This is where the somatic connection begins. It's not just about remembering. It's about *feeling* again—through your body, not just your thoughts.

This step may bring tears, laughter, longing, or joy. Let it. You are not analyzing the song; you are letting it awaken parts of you that have been silent.

STEP 4: CULL AND CURATE

Your first list may have 25 or 50 songs. That's beautiful. But when you're ready, start narrowing to the 15 or so that hold the most resonance. Choose the ones that feel like a *homecoming*.

Ask yourself:

- Does this song still live in my body?
- Is this moment essential to my story?

STEP 5: LISTEN WITHOUT DOING

This is the most important part.

Make a date with yourself. Go to a place where you feel safe, calm, and open. Put on your playlist and listen. No scrolling. No folding laundry. No podcast in the background.

Let the songs move through you. Let them break things open or settle things down. Pay attention to:

- Where in your body the music lands
- Any unexpected memories that arise
- Physical sensations, like warmth, tingling, tightness, or release

This is somatic wisdom in action. Your body holds your life story. Music lets you hear it.

STEP 6: REFLECT AND RECORD

Once you've listened, write down what came up. You can do this song-by-song or as a stream-of-consciousness journaling session. Some questions to guide you:

- What did I remember that I'd forgotten?
- What am I grieving?
- What am I reclaiming?
- What part of me feels more alive now?

This reflection isn't about closure; it's about awareness. Awareness opens the door to reconnection and evolution.

OPTIONAL: SHARE IN COMMUNITY

This practice can be deeply personal, but also incredibly powerful when shared. If it feels right, invite a friend or a group to do it with you. Create a space where you each play a song, share a memory, and witness one another without judgment.

You may find, like I did, that your story helps others hear their own more clearly.

WHY IT WORKS

You might be wondering—*why music? Why now?*

Because music roots memory in the body. And as humans, especially in midlife, we're often cut off from that body. Years of caretaking, chronic stress, menopause, trauma—these all create disconnection. We live from the neck up.

Music gently leads us back down. It bypasses the inner critic and awakens sensation, memory, and truth.

There's a reason the songs that hit hardest often come from our adolescence. We were more embodied then. Our sensory gates were wide open. And when we return to those songs now, we return to the parts of us we left behind.

FINAL INVITATION

Your life deserves a soundtrack. One that isn't curated by a marketing team or an algorithm. One that tells *your* story, in *your* voice.

So here's your invitation:

- Create a playlist of 15 songs that tell the story of you.
- Sit with each song. Let it show you what it needs to.
- Listen with your whole body.
- Write, reflect, and—if you're ready—share.

If this process lit something up in you, I'd love to hear about it. There's magic in this because your voice has been playing all along.

It just needed you to *press play.*

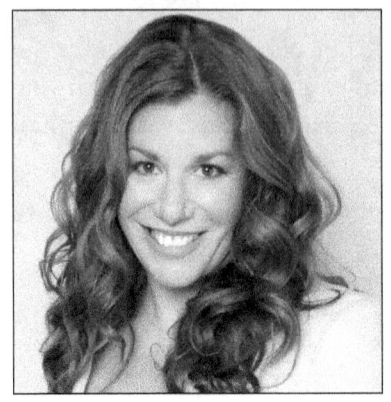

Lisa Boate is the founder of *Liberated Menopause Consulting & Coaching*, host of the *Transforming 45* podcast, and a passionate advocate for creating menopause empowered workplaces. After more than two decades as an educator navigating systems that often felt too rigid for real transformation, she stepped away from the institution to help women—and the organizations they work in—reclaim their voices, their power, and their well-being in midlife.

Based in London, Ontario, Lisa lives with her husband, their two brilliant young humans (when they are home from University), and their two very spicy dogs, Lola and Gemma. When she's not coaching, creating, or recording, you'll find her hosting kitchen dance parties to the best of the 80s and 90s, baking bread, jumping in the pool, or strolling by the river. She believes midlife isn't a crisis—it's an invitation to get loud and groove to the music of our own bodies in new and exciting ways.

Connect with Lisa

>Website: https://www.liberatedmenopause.ca/
>Email: lisa@liberatedmenopause.ca
>Instagram: https://www.instagram.com/lboate/
>LinkedIn: https://bit.ly/3ZHZcER
>Podcast: https://bit.ly/44H7gaB
>YouTube: https://www.youtube.com/@Transforming45/featured
>TikTok: https://www.tiktok.com/@lisaboate
>Free Gift: https://pages.lisaboate.com/free-guide-1
>*Your Life as A Sound Track* Journal: https://amzn.to/45wcBU9
>*Transforming 45* Playlist Episode: https://bit.ly/3U3V7Y0

CHAPTER 13

Guided by Grace

A Journey Through Surrender and Acceptance

Tina Green

MY STORY

Agh! Why won't she stop crying?

I pace the room, bouncing my newborn, trying everything I know to soothe her. But the screaming continues—a piercing, relentless sound that echoes through my entire body. She looks like a screaming tomato: red-faced, scrunched, furious. My whole body clenches.

She's been changed and fed. Maybe she's tired. Why won't she settle down?

I'll sing "You Are My Sunshine" for her.

I sang it over and over, but still, she cried.

I feel like a complete failure. I can't even soothe my baby. Something must be wrong. What is she trying to tell me? I need to take her to the doctor.

My first daughter, Grace, was born slightly premature, a tiny but mighty four pounds. She fully developed in every way, but without body fat, she couldn't maintain her temperature. We stayed in the hospital together for eight days, and right from the start, my experience as a mother was a rocky one.

I walked into motherhood with incredibly rigid ideas of how I'd raise my child. It was going to be different—even better—than how I was raised. I created a detailed birth plan, hired a doula to advocate for a natural birth on my terms, and envisioned myself breastfeeding, using cloth diapers, avoiding all toxic baby products, and co-sleeping to form an unshakable bond.

None of it went the way I planned. Not one bit. And in my mind, that translated to absolute failure. I sank into a deep postpartum depression. A tearful conversation with my husband went something like this:

"I'm such a failure; I can't do this. You and Grace would be better off without me."

"Tina, that's not true. This isn't you. We need to get you some help."

And he was right. I knew I needed help. I cried and cried and cried, and then immediately found a therapist in my town. Over just a few sessions, she helped me come back to myself through Eye Movement Desensitization and Reprocessing (EMDR) therapy, a therapy that helps people heal from the emotional distress of upsetting or traumatic experiences.

Once I felt like myself again, a powerful truth surfaced: I couldn't control my child, nor was I meant to.

As soon as those words left my mouth, my next move became very clear to me. *I need to surrender. I need to meet her where she is, not where I expect her to be.* I immediately felt the tension leave me like a full-body sigh of relief.

That rocky beginning as a mother became my first profound lesson in surrender. I always say Grace is my biggest teacher. I was finally ready to accept that I had a healthy baby who simply needed to scream, and she needed me to be with her in that scream. She needed me to accept her as she was and show her she was safe, even in her most distressing moments.

I stopped fighting her cries. I stopped trying to fix her. Instead, I started giving her a daily bath followed by a massage. When she cried, I stayed calm and held her close, no longer fixated on stopping the screaming, but just being present with her. Once I truly surrendered to her needs and accepted her as a healthy baby who needed to use her voice, everything started getting better.

She still went from zero to 60 very fast, but my calm presence quickly calmed her down, and the connection we created through the daily massages also helped a lot.

Wow, surrender was exactly what I needed to do. The way I acted made it worse. It feels good not to struggle.

Finally, at three months old, Grace even started smiling. Her sweet smile felt like the most incredible reward. I ran to my husband. "She smiled! She smiled! Come and see!"

While this was my first conscious experience of surrender and acceptance, it quickly became a powerful, guiding practice in my life.

Looking back, that intense struggle was driven mainly by perfectionism and avoidance. My perfectionism had me trying to control everything around me, from her birth to her temperament, in order to feel okay. I needed things to be perfect so I could be perfect. Instead of truly being present with her, I was consumed by my reaction to her crying and my fear of failure.

This perfectionism was highly rewarded in my career, where my relentless drive for perfection often meant hitting impossible deadlines and achieving seemingly unattainable goals. Not surprisingly, I carried that same demanding expectation into parenting and my marriage. What an unrealistic burden I placed on everyone, especially myself! I now realize that as I strived to be the perfect mother, I subtly expected my daughter to be perfect, too. The same held for my marriage. It was a profound lesson I needed to learn to move forward successfully in my relationships—and Grace, in her beautiful yet challenging way, was the one to teach me.

It turned out some of what she displayed as an infant was simply her temperament, which continued to manifest throughout her childhood. Over the years, she consistently invited me to surrender and accept, gently nudging me beyond my need for control.

What I know now is that even if every single thing in my plan had come true, it wasn't going to make me feel okay. Because that underlying fear and perfectionism would still exist, and they'd only grow bigger, continually showing up and demanding I react to them.

Surrendering, I've learned, often requires me to get honest with myself—to step out of denial and admit the truth. I have to acknowledge what I avoid or cling to. That's where true surrender begins.

When challenging situations come up, I often remember that initial lesson from Grace: *Oh right, at this point there's nothing I can do to make this better, so I'm going to surrender. I'll stop trying to fix it and see what happens.* Sure enough, the situation improves, and my internal struggle comes to an end.

What I didn't fully grasp then was that surrender was more than just a successful "tool"; it was the very key to unlocking a deeper spiritual path within me.

Years later, I was invited on an author's journey to Mexico—an experience that deepened everything I learned about surrender and revealed an even deeper acceptance.

One of our excursions was a visit to the Basilica of Our Lady of Guadalupe, located close to the site where, in the early 1500s, Mother Mary reportedly appeared several times to a humble man named Juan Diego.

She asked Juan Diego to convince the bishop to build a church on that site. To prove her appearance, she caused roses to bloom out of season, and when he gathered them in his cloak, an image of her miraculously appeared on the fabric. Because of her, many indigenous people embraced the Catholic church rather than face death, the choice presented by the Catholic Spaniards. The story is rich with symbolism, particularly for the blending of cultures and beliefs, representing a new birth and a pathway to peace amidst brutal colonialism.

This sacred cloak, the tilma, hangs prominently in the basilica, and we headed inside to see it. The invitation to enter the basilica triggered my resistance. You see, this was a Catholic church, and I carried deep resentment from my fear-based upbringing within Catholicism. I wanted nothing to do with going inside. I was only convinced by one of my co-authors, who happened to be an expert on all things Our Lady of Guadalupe, to try to separate her spirit from the institution.

"Focus on her spirit as the universal mother and see if you can separate her spirit from the church," she urged.

Okay, I can do this. I can focus on her and not the church. I can approach this with curiosity.

I didn't know it yet, but that decision to surrender, to release my resistance and step through those doors, was the beginning of a profound spiritual awakening for me.

As I stood before the almost 500-year-old sacred tilma, an intense feeling of love rose within my body. It became even more intense as we visited her chapel at the top of the hill where she first appeared. I was filled with such overwhelming love that I was disoriented, not fully understanding what was happening.

Later that night, I participated in Sacred Journey Breathwork. During the session, I went on a profound inner journey. Our Lady of Guadalupe came to me, and I was an infant in her arms. She held me close and fed me from her breast. I felt so safe and loved, a feeling I had never experienced so completely before. As she held me, the world swirled around us like a chaotic, furious wind. There were visions of war, my mother and father, children playing, a child crying alone, animals dancing, and my mother crying.

I feel so safe and so full of love.

While the chaos of the world swirled around us, I suckled her breast, drinking in her love and nourishment, and she gazed steadily into my eyes. As the baby, I had no awareness of the chaos, but as the journeyer, I was the witness. I could see all the turmoil, yet from the safety of her embrace, I experienced a profound detachment from the suffering.

The love is overwhelming. She is my spiritual mother.

It was a profoundly moving experience, bringing forth both tears of joy and grief. I was so joyful to have so clearly found my spiritual mother, a connection that felt incredibly real. This allowed me to release a significant amount of grief that had lived inside me over my relationship with my human mother.

Then, I truly understood surrender was not just a tool; it was an integral part of my spiritual practice. When I surrender, release my resistance, and let go of suffering, love flows through me effortlessly.

From this point on, my spirituality became my path to healing. On this path, I learned to love and accept myself without changing anything about myself.

I welcomed the Christ consciousness back into my life, a sacred and profound story I detailed in another Brave Healer publication, *Shaman Heart: We Are the Ones We've Been Waiting For,* and I experienced immense relief through surrender every day. I took up daily prayer, surrendering to a higher power, which for me is God.

I now understand, more clearly than ever, that I don't have control. Trying to force outcomes only creates suffering for me and for those I love. Surrender is a daily practice I'm dedicated to, as it allows me to lead a freer, more joyful life. I don't have to try to be happy, I just am. If I find myself unhappy, I know it's an invitation to surrender.

In every case when I decide to surrender a challenge or an unknown to God, I also surrender the outcome and ask for guidance.

For example, I struggled with speaking my truth in a challenging relationship with my boss and the founder of the organization I worked for, which had a large community I loved deeply. I risked giving up my leadership and involvement in that community. The relationship dynamic as it stood was unacceptable to me, and my life became unmanageable. I had to surrender both the challenging relationship and the outcome. The surrender wouldn't be effective if I still clung to the outcome, so I surrendered both. It was a difficult decision, and it took months for me to come to terms with it and fully surrender. I'm so grateful I took a stand for myself.

I feel immense relief since fully surrendering. I left that position, learned valuable lessons, and have maintained many of the relationships I cherish. This experience allowed me to devote more energy to my personal pursuits, so in the end, I was guided back to myself, and my life is now more manageable.

An example where I didn't surrender the outcome was during the pandemic. My family had significant struggles. Grace and her younger sister were stuck at home in virtual school, and Grace struggled with the isolation and online learning. My husband was depressed, and my work as the program director at a local nonprofit tripled in volume. Something had to give.

In this case, I surrendered the challenge but not the outcome, and it was a hard struggle. I decided to take a leave of absence from my work, and I had a picture of what it would look like when I returned. The decision to take a nine-month break from my job was a huge relief to me and my family; however, when I returned, my temporary replacement was permanent, and she was now my boss. That, I could handle, but she didn't trust me with all the staff I hired and the systems I created that helped shape the organization. It was hard, and I eventually resigned, feeling betrayed and bitter. I struggled with it for many months. I believe if I had surrendered the outcome, I would've moved through the struggle more quickly.

At the time of writing this chapter, Grace again invites me to surrender as she's about to fly away to New York City to attend the performing arts college of her dreams. This is a big one that has already begun, with lots of joy and grief. I surrender every day, and I trust she's well-prepared for life on her own. She knows I'll always be available to support her.

Every time I surrender, I learn a valuable lesson. This practice continues to shape how I live, love, and lead, moment by moment. While it isn't always easy, the path of surrender is always liberating.

THE TOOL

"Listen to this truth: We are each in our present circumstances for a reason. There is a lesson, a valuable lesson, that must be learned before we can move forward".

~ Melodie Beattie, *The Language of Letting Go*

I'm excited to share my process of coming to surrender, though first, I want to admit I'm not perfect at this. I'm human. I have things coming up all the time, and I've become more adept at recognizing when I try to control a situation and need to surrender. It's a practice, and no human is perfect at it.

When you feel yourself struggling, use the prompts below to help guide you into a state of surrender. You can write your answers in a journal, speak them aloud, or simply reflect.

- Who am I trying to control right now?
- How does it serve me if I let go?
- How does it serve them if I let go?
- What am I afraid will happen if I let go?
- What might happen if I surrendered this, just for today?

When you're ready to surrender, I suggest a prayer or meditation as follows:

Thank you, God (or Divine Feminine, Great Spirit, Universe, Beloved), for my breath and another day of life, and for the ways you guide me and provide unconditional love.

Today, I want to surrender to you *[state your issue or relationship]*.

I surrender my fear and my need to control.

Please help me to be honest with myself, see clearly, and let go.

I place this situation in your care.

I release the outcome. I choose peace.

Please lead me with your wisdom.

Please guide me on how to move forward.

Please fill me with your love.

I surrender, and I trust.

Amen. And so it is.

If you find it very hard to surrender, you might need to do it multiple times before you feel the relief of true surrender. Some things take weeks or months of daily prayer to truly release.

It's not about perfection. It's about commitment.

The path of surrender isn't always easy, but it's always liberating. Each time I lay something down, I make space to rise higher—guided not by control, but by trust.

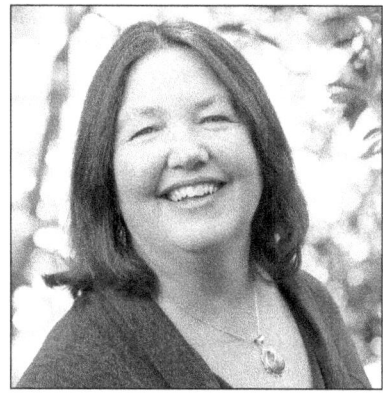

Tina Green brings her devoted and loving mother energy to everyone she serves. In her safe, welcoming presence, she helps your vulnerability, voice, and wisdom emerge from hiding.

She guides and witnesses you as you navigate shame, fear, low self-esteem, and codependency, so you can learn to use your voice, prioritize yourself, and love and accept yourself unconditionally. Tina's signature program, The Art of Putting Yourself First, is presented in person throughout the United States and online via Zoom. She also leads powerful self-love retreats in awe-inspiring places around the world, and she co-facilitates the potent, year-long program, Toltec Medicine Wheel of Transformation, in Northern California.

Tina's service is deeply informed by her lived experience recovering from profound codependency, shame, fear, and low self-esteem. She now fully loves and accepts herself, and she is passionate about guiding others on their experiential journey to self-love and acceptance.

Tina is the #1 bestselling author of *The Life-Changing Power of Self-Love: An Essential Guide* and the founder of Exposing the Roots. She's a master transformational facilitator of the healing arts, an ordained minister, a certified celebrant, and a Toltec Sacred Journey Breathwork Facilitator. She apprenticed at the master level with Jeremy Pajer and Stephanie Urbina Jones of Freedom Folk & Soul.

With 20 years of experience as an executive in nonprofit and financial services, Tina also holds certifications in life coaching and massage therapy, and she's a holistic chef.

Tina lives in Northern California with her husband, two teenage daughters, two dogs, and a cat. She loves to be in nature, garden, cook, travel, and experience live music and theater.

Join Tina's free "Women's Self-Love Community" for inspiration and access to complimentary self-love events:
https://www.facebook.com/groups/theselflovecommunity

Connect with Tina:

Website: https://www.ExposingTheRoots.com

Email: Tina@ExposingTheRoots.com

Substack: https://substack.com/@selflovequeen

Instagram: https://www.instagram.com/ExposingTheRoots

Facebook: https://www.facebook.com/ExposingTheRoots

LinkedIn: https://www.linkedin.com/in/exposingtheroots/

CHAPTER 14

The Great Allowing

The Liberation of Doing Less and Trusting More

Patty Nagle, LMHC, Grof Breathwork Facilitator

To my dear mother, Joan Louise Nagle, who navigated the Greatest of the Great Allowing by passing on July 8, 2025—just after I completed this chapter.
Mom, you were my inspiration, my anchor, and most of all, my beloved mother.
I love you to the moon and back.

MY STORY

WHAT IS HEALING?

Did you ever stop to ask yourself, "What is healing?"

As I considered writing this chapter, I asked myself, "How would I define healing?" The answer came quickly and clearly: Healing is any step I take that moves me toward wholeness. It's anything that restores balance, increases my awareness of the aspects of myself that reside in the unconscious, and makes me a better human being.

The healing process can take many forms. It can be sudden and dramatic—a lightning bolt sparked by a life-threatening diagnosis, the death of a loved one, or the collapse of a cherished relationship. But healing can also unfold slowly, subtly, almost imperceptibly.

My healing is a long, spiraling journey toward wholeness. Only when I pause and look back do I realize how far I've come. I have healed; I've changed; I'm a different person; I'm more whole.

Persistent curiosity fuels my journey—an inner questioning about whether there might be more to life, more to being human, than what I was taught to believe. A thirst to learn and challenge limitations drove me, whether they were imposed by others or self-inflicted. Time and again, healing invited me to step beyond my comfort zone. After all, most transformation begins outside one's comfort zone.

THE CULTURE OF DOING

To understand my path, you need to know a bit about how I was raised: I was encouraged to be a "doing machine." In my family of origin, doing more was rewarded, and stillness was frowned upon. Productivity equaled love. My mother, a woman whose approval I craved, was happiest when I was doing. It didn't matter what I was doing, so long as I was doing something. And so, I became someone who tried harder, did more, and never paused to question if there was any other way.

Nothing illustrates my upbringing around the pressure to always be *doing* quite like this funny story.

During one of my mother's visits to see me in Santa Fe, she drove me to work and picked me up later that day. On our ride home, in an attempt to make conversation, I asked her, "How was your day?"

She responded by listing all the things she did for me since we parted ways that morning.

Then I asked her, "How were the girls?" referring to my two dogs who stayed home with her.

"They're good, but all they do is lie around." It took me a moment to let what she just said sink in as she continued with her report. "So, I finally went over to them and told them to go outside and find something to do!"

Again, I had to let what she said sink in. After a few moments and in disbelief, I said, "You what?"

She replied, "I told them to get outside and find something to do because it's not healthy for them to be lying around all day."

By this time, I had started to feel a bit defensive. "Mom, that's what dogs do!" I countered. "They have big fur coats, so they lie around especially when it's hot out!"

It evoked a familiar feeling in my body of what I experienced growing up. That is what she constantly said to me and my three siblings: "Go out and find something to do, or I'll find something for you to do!"

It hit me like a ton of bricks!

To this day, that story saves me years of trying to explain my mother to a therapist! I can now laugh at that story, and it always gets a good laugh when I tell it.

As the oldest of four, I took on the unofficial role of Mom's best overachiever. I found a powerful channel for my energy in sports. I loved them, and I excelled. It also pleased my mother and garnered her attention because she was very athletic for a woman of her time.

As a young adult, I funneled my drive into running road races, which led to triathlons. By my early 30s, I completed six Ironman triathlons and ran marathons as "training runs." I lived by the belief that "where there's a will, there's a way," and with enough will, anything was possible. And it was, for a time.

Don't get me wrong, this period was transformative. I learned that most limitations are illusions. I experienced firsthand the human potential to achieve, to endure, to grow. But over time, the constant striving left me drained. I was out of balance. I began to question the compulsion to push and prove. I longed for a change, though I didn't yet know what form it would take.

I share my story because I suspect many people reach a similar point in their lives, feeling exhausted and out of balance. Let's face it, our American culture values doing, knowing, controlling, and managing. My obsession was physical, but for someone else, it might have been their career, their body, or their children.

Whatever it might be, we're often left believing we need to make things happen, do more, and try harder. We need to manage other people, our bodies, our children, our own emotions, and perhaps even other people's emotions. Often, feeling overwhelmed, we reach a tipping point.

A TIPPING POINT IN THE DESERT

My tipping point came in the mid-1990s, when I participated in a modern-day vision quest: a four-day solo fast in the desert, hosted by Upaya, a Buddhist retreat center in Santa Fe, New Mexico. True to form, I approached it with grit and determination, intent on enduring and overcoming.

But something unexpected happened. The facilitators encouraged me to slow down, to relinquish the pursuit.

This opportunity wasn't about doing more and pushing; in fact, that approach could be dangerous in such a context and make me a liability.

For the first time, I encountered the stillness of simply being. Alone in the wilderness, free of tasks and expectations, I began to listen. To notice. To breathe. To soften. By the end of my four-day solo, I didn't want to come back; it felt like I had truly "come home."

This experience was a turning point. Upon reflection, I can say it was my first experience of what I eventually referred to as, "The Great Allowing."

I connected with my feminine essence—rooted in receptivity, openness, and presence—which felt like stepping into a more whole version of myself. The natural world, vast and quiet, mirrored back the presence I ignored in myself.

I started to realize that doing more and trying harder wasn't the only way forward.

REWIRING FROM WITHIN: HEALING THROUGH EXPANDED STATES OF CONSCIOUSNESS (ESC)

The sheer vastness and beauty of the Southwest tugged at something deep in me, and I felt compelled to move west. After leaving New England, the environment that shaped me, I questioned the "try harder" mentality at a deeper level. Seeking a new way of being, I was introduced to expanded states of consciousness (ESC) work through psychedelics and Holotropic (Grof) breathwork. These tools became essential to my healing.

In the field of psychedelic healing, there's a concept known as the Default Mode Network (DMN). This refers to the deeply ingrained neural pathways that govern our beliefs, thoughts, relational patterns, and behaviors. These patterns often form early on in our lives as a way of adapting to the environment we're in. Until we become aware of our DMNs, we usually stay stuck in those neurobiological ruts, making change difficult. This is the potential of ESC work: it can reveal what has been unconscious, and invites us into new ways of being.

Through ESC work, I became aware of my DMN: the compulsive doing, the self-management, the striving. My first taste of stillness, I experienced during my time in nature, awakened something in me.

ESC work invited me further into this space—to feel, to allow, to witness without needing to fix. I began to see the consequences of my lifelong need to control, manage, and push. I experienced those consequences in my body as tightness and a subtle hypervigilance.

The ESC work brought me to explore the concept of surrender and what that meant. My associations were strong; surrender implied failure, giving up, and losing.

But I was on to something. I began to sense a deeper intelligence guiding me—one that didn't come from my mind or brain, but from a deeper place: the psyche. This knowing led me to the concept and practice of allowing.

Allowing carried none of the resistance that surrender evoked. It felt softer, more accepting to me.

As my awareness grew, so did my capacity to choose differently. I formed new neural pathways grounded more in trust, spaciousness, and presence. This shift opened a door to profound healing. Through allowing, I created space for those shifts. I permitted myself to rewire from the inside out.

THE PRACTICE OF ALLOWING

In ESC work, I learned that healing arises when we remain open and receptive to whatever shows up. This was the exact medicine for my goal-oriented, driven personality. In allowing, I found balance.

Over time, the practice of allowing became central to my path. It emerged again and again in expanded states and during integration.

The more I allowed, the more I trusted. I experienced a freedom I never knew. I didn't always have to be in control. I didn't need to know everything. I could rest in something larger than myself.

Allowing showed me that presence is powerful. It taught me to meet each moment without forcing outcomes. It reminded me that healing doesn't come from effort alone, but from surrendering to life's natural unfolding.

As this healing process deepened, the name for what I experienced became clear: The Great Allowing.

THE PRACTICE OF ALLOWING IN DAILY LIFE

You don't need to engage in ESC work, such as psychedelics or breathwork, to begin allowing. Opportunities exist every day.

Perhaps it's at work, where you resist the urge to manage a situation and let it unfold instead. Maybe it's at home, where you give space to a partner or child to step into a new role. Perhaps it's with yourself, choosing to pause rather than push.

These acts can empower you and others to step up in different ways of responding to a given situation.

Allowing isn't passive. It's an active, conscious choice. It asks us to slow down, stay awake to our patterned way of being, and trust. It invites us to listen deeply, to stay awake and curious, and to befriend the unknown or unfamiliar.

This isn't easy work. Most of us were taught that control is strength and productivity is virtue. But true strength often lies in restraint. And true freedom can come from surrender, or just allowing.

LIVING THE GREAT ALLOWING

The Great Allowing isn't a destination. It's a practice, a return, a breath-by-breath commitment to presence. It challenges the deeply rooted belief that we must do more, manage outcomes, or know everything in advance.

When we allow, we enter the field of possibility. We discover the magic that emerges when we release control and open to what wants to unfold. In a culture that idolizes doing, allowing is a radical act.

So no, allowing doesn't mean "doing nothing." It means recognizing the moments when doing less creates space for more. It means choosing trust over control, curiosity over certainty, and presence over performance.

For me, learning to allow is a powerful part of my healing, guiding me closer to a sense of wholeness. For you, it may be the first step into unknown terrain, full of mystery and possibility.

I invite you to join me in the unfolding, in the discomfort, in the grace—in the profound, life-changing practice of The Great Allowing.

THE TOOL

Embracing The Great Allowing is an ongoing commitment—a practice of choosing presence over pressure, trust over control. Below are a few tools to support you on this path. I hope you allow them to serve you and encourage you to take what you need, leave the rest.

JOURNAL PROMPTS

Choose one or two questions that resonate. Let your writing be honest, unfiltered, and spacious.

- Where in my life am I trying hard to control an outcome? What would it feel like to try less and trust more?
- What patterns or beliefs was I raised with about productivity and self-worth? How do they still show up today?
- When was the last time I paused before reacting? What did I notice in that space?

- What might I discover if I allow myself to not know, for just a moment?

- What part of me resists slowing down, and what does that part need to feel safe?

- If I stopped managing everything for one day, what do I fear might happen? And what might happen?

REFLECTION QUESTIONS

Use these to identify your "healing edge"— the tender, growing places where your capacity to allow evolves.

- What does *wholeness* mean to me right now?

- Can I recall a time I allowed instead of pushed, and something beautiful emerged?

- In what situations do I most often override my inner knowing or intuition?

- Who in my life models the energy of allowing? What can I learn from them?

- What do I believe I must "do" to be loved? Where did that belief begin?

SIMPLE PRACTICES FOR DAILY LIFE

Small, consistent practices build the capacity to allow.

- The Pause Practice. Once a day, when you feel the urge to act, speak, or fix, pause. Take three slow breaths. Ask: *Is action needed here, or is this an opportunity to allow?*

- Mindful Unknowing. At least once this week, sit with a life question *without* trying to answer it. Let it breathe. Let it unfold.

- Body Engagement. Set a timer once per day to pause and ask: What does my body need right now? *What does my soul need right now?* Listen. No judgment. Just allow.

- Do Less, Notice More. Choose one task or conversation to approach with less doing and more presence. Notice what changes. Let yourself be surprised.

- The Great Allowing Hour. Block one hour this week with no plans, goals, or obligations. Let it be an open space. Afterward, journal: *What surfaced when I allowed space?*

Here's to The Great Allowing and our capacity to trust in something greater than ourselves to support our individual and collective healing.

For more support, resources, and inspiration, visit www.thegreatallowing.com. If you'd like to reach me, please submit the contact form on my website. I'd love to hear from you.

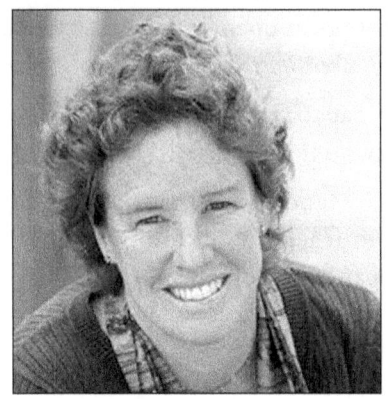

Patty Nagle is a licensed mental health counselor (LMHC), certified Grof® Breathwork facilitator, and expanded states of consciousness consultant. She supports individuals navigating the complex, beautiful, and often bewildering terrain of healing and transformation. She specializes in helping people prepare for and integrate expanded states of consciousness, including psychedelic experiences, offering grounded, heart-centered guidance for those on the path of inner exploration.

Patty's approach is rooted in transpersonal and Jungian psychology, deep listening, and a deep respect for the fact that the healing process rarely follows a straight line. Before becoming a therapist, she spent many years in nonprofit management, a background that continues to inform her work with a grounded, practical lens and a strong attunement to both personal and collective well-being.

Today, Patty brings together professional expertise and intuitive presence to create spaces where clients feel safe to unravel, release, and rediscover themselves. Her work honors the wisdom of the psyche and is guided by a quiet trust in the human capacity to heal when given the space and support to do so naturally. Whether working one-on-one or facilitating group experiences, Patty invites trust, curiosity, and surrender to the inner knowing that lives within each of us.

She lives in a small village just north of Santa Fe, New Mexico, where the high desert landscape offers both inspiration and solace. Surrounded by nature and accompanied by her two beloved dogs, Patty finds renewal in the simplicity of daily life and the beauty of the natural world. Her writing and work reflect a lifelong curiosity about the human experience— and a devotion to the quiet wisdom that emerges when we learn to try less and trust more.

Connect with Patty:
Website: http://www.thegreatallowing.com/

CHAPTER 15

When the Therapist Breaks

Healing Burnout with Ecstatic Dance

Dr. Tiffany McBride, DSPS, LCPC

MY STORY

Oh shit, I need to walk.

It was already too late in the morning, but I promised myself I'd move today. I didn't hydrate. I wasn't prepared. But I went anyway.

"Just go," I told myself. "You need this. You said you would."

So, I stepped outside, not knowing how hot the midwestern sun in June would bear down on me.

The first stretch felt good—about 30 minutes in, and I felt strong. My body moved. My mind cleared. I thought, *See? You needed this. You're fine.*

But then I turned around, and it was like all the heat waited for me, just around the corner. My heart started beating fast. Too fast. My skin grew flushed and sticky. My head felt light. I told myself to slow down, but everything inside me sped up. As I turned onto the final street toward my house, dizziness slammed into me. I had to stop. My legs shook.

"Oh no," I whispered. "Not right now. We're not doing this. We are not doing this right now."

I put one foot in front of the other. Slower. *Just keep going.*

And that's when the song came on: "Never Say Die" by Neoni. And I swear it was like the soundtrack to my stubbornness, a war cry in the form of music. Heavy, cinematic, defiant. It felt like it was written for moments like this, when you're crawling to the finish line. When you're empty but still pushing, because why? Because you said you would?

I started to feel high, like my body wasn't entirely mine anymore. My vision blurred, and I kept repeating to myself, "Almost there. Almost there. You're almost home."

It was like a movie. The dehydrated woman, sweat-soaked and stumbling up a mountain she didn't plan to climb, whispering mantras to keep her body moving.

"Just get home. Once I get there, it'll be okay."

And then, another voice:

But why do I always have to make it feel like this? Why do I always wait until I'm on the verge of collapse to listen? Why do I push myself to the edge and then act surprised when my body screams? Why does everything feel like a test I have to pass to earn rest?

This walk wasn't just about heat exhaustion. This was burnout, a physical embodiment of how I've lived most of my life: overheated, overextended, and undernourished. Doing too much. Ignoring the early signs. Convincing myself I can make it if I just keep going.

Whispering, "Almost there," like it's some kind of reward.

I told Natalie about the walk later that night on a video call.

I sat on my porch, the air finally cooling, iced tea sweating in my hand. My body still felt a little shaky, as if it hadn't fully recovered.

"I think I actually gave myself heat exhaustion," I said, half-laughing, half-dead serious.

"Oh no," she said. "Are you okay?"

"I mean, yeah, physically. But it hit me hard. Not just the heat; it was something deeper. Like, this is my life. This is what I keep doing. Pushing too hard until I crash."

"You mean the burnout?" she asked, already knowing.

"Yeah." I sighed. "I've clinically burnt out so many times over the years as a psychotherapist, but I always just changed something—my role, my job, the setting. I thought that would fix it. I thought I could keep going if I kept reinventing the path."

"But you were still walking the same way," she said gently.

I sipped my tea and then added, "The truth is, burnout isn't about the job. It's about how I've been carrying it all—my own trauma, my own suffering, and trying to help others fix theirs. It's a lot."

Natalie asked me carefully, "Can anyone get burned out, even if they aren't a helping professional?"

I blurted without hesitation. "Yes. Absolutely."

"Even you?" she asked. "You love helping people. You've always been the strong one."

I laughed. "That's exactly why I'm burnt out. Because I keep pushing. I keep helping. I keep showing up until I have nothing left."

She was quiet. "So, what does it feel like? Burnout?"

"It's not always dramatic. It's not panic attacks or crying in the bathroom, though I've had those, too. Sometimes it's just dread. It's waking up and feeling like your soul has been sucked out of you in your sleep. It's looking at your calendar and feeling like you're being slowly crushed by obligations that used to light you up."

"Damn."

"It's like your joy gets muted. Your spark dims. But you keep going because that's what you do. And then one day, a walk in the sun takes you out, and you realize you've been walking dehydrated for years."

Natalie sat with that. "So, is that why you're taking the sabbatical?"

"Yeah," I said, exhaling. "It's finally time. I kept thinking I could heal while holding everything together. But I can't. I had to put it down."

She looked at me through the screen with so much tenderness. "That's brave, you know."

I smiled, feeling the weight of it settle into truth. "I don't feel brave. I feel tired. But for the first time in a long time, I also feel honest." I paused. "And the truth is, this burnout is leading to physical issues too."

She leaned in. "What do you mean?"

I hesitated. Took a long sip. "I didn't tell you, but I had a doctor's appointment a few days ago."

Her face softened with concern. "What happened?"

I exhaled slowly. "Let's just say I got a full-on come-to-geezus talk. My doctor looked me dead in the eyes and said, 'You're going to have a major health crisis if you don't make changes. Soon.'"

Natalie's eyes widened. "Whoa."

"Yeah. It wasn't subtle. The doctor wasn't sugarcoating anything. And I think I needed that. My body has been screaming at me for a while, but I kept ignoring it. I kept saying, I'm fine, I'm strong, I'll rest later." I looked down at my tea. "But later doesn't always come."

"What did you do?"

"I cut my caseload in half. I finally admitted I couldn't keep showing up for everyone else if I wasn't showing up for myself. I've been canceling some things, saying no. Even taking naps." I smiled a little. "It still feels weird. Like I'm doing something wrong."

"You're not," Natalie said. "You're doing something necessary."

"I know," I said. "But it's hard. I've spent my whole life proving I can carry it all. But now? I don't want to carry it like that anymore."

We sat in silence for a few moments.

"I just—I don't want my body to be the price I pay for being useful," I finally said.

Natalie's voice was soft but firm. "Then don't. You've already given so much. Maybe it's time to give some of that back to yourself."

The next morning, I sat at the kitchen table, staring at my planner, fingers grazing the pages like they were sacred texts. Color-coded boxes. Notes scribbled in the margins. Post-its layered on top of each other like a Jenga tower of obligation.

Technically, I was on a part-time "sabbatical." But my planner told a different story.

I stared at the packed week ahead: "Create workshop outline," "Schedule content shoot," "Build a website," "Follow up on retreat list," "Respond to so-and-so's email." The tasks went on.

None of the tasks mentioned "rest" or "have fun."

The kettle hissed behind me. I turned it off, poured myself a cup of tea, and sat back down.

And then I just stared. The guilt crept in like a fog.

Why haven't you done any of this? You're wasting time. Other people would kill for this freedom and look at you, floundering.

I slammed the planner shut. Too loud. The tea rippled in the mug.

I pushed back from the table and wandered into the living room, arms crossed like I was trying to hold myself in.

I paced. Then I paused. Then I crumpled onto the floor, cross-legged and tense.

"I don't know how to rest," I whispered aloud. The words caught in my throat like they weren't meant to be said.

I sat in silence for a long time. And it wasn't peaceful. It was itchy. Confrontational.

I don't want to sit in this. I don't want to be alone in the mess. I don't want to hear the deeper voice underneath all the doing.

So, I stood up. Walked over to my speaker. Turned it on. Let the first song that came up play. A beat dropped. Slow, sensual, familiar. Without thinking, I let my body move.

A sway at first. Then, a small spiral in my hips. Then my arms rose, slow and liquid until I was dancing, not to perform, but to release.

No one was watching. No one needed anything from me. There was no outcome attached. Just movement.

And in the rhythm, I started to remember.

I used to dance like this all the time.

Tears welled up—not from sadness, but from recognition. This was what "rest" looked like for me. Not stillness in bed, spiraling in my mind. Not empty space filled with guilt. But movement that brought me back to myself, to my body.

For years, I wasn't fully present in my body. During the COVID years, it felt like everything fragmented. My work, my routines, my relationships, my sense of safety. I lived in my head, producing, spiraling, surviving.

I adapted. I created. I held space for others. But somewhere in all of it, I lost touch with myself. My body became the background noise; something to manage, ignore, silence.

Just get through the day. Just do the thing. Just focus on the next task.

I didn't breathe deeply. I didn't eat. I didn't stretch. I didn't listen. I became a mind with a task list. A nervous system on autopilot.

I danced to two songs. Maybe three. By the time I stopped, something shifted.

My planner was still closed. My tea was cold. But for the first time in days, my breath was deep. My body wasn't tense. I felt alive.

In the days that followed, my schedule opened up. The emails slowed. The calendar had gaps. There was less to do, which should have felt like a relief. Sometimes it did. But other times, it didn't.

I woke up and felt this strange, unsettled pull to *fill the space*. I started piling the day with "fun" things—art, writing, vision boards, half-baked business plans—not because I needed to, but because I didn't know what to do with the quiet.

It was like productivity was my favorite drug, just repackaged in prettier colors. And then the next day would hit. Exhaustion. Again.

I found myself sleeping in, staring out windows, caught in loops that felt more like spirals than insights. And that's when the thoughts came in—the sharp-edged ones.

What are you even doing? You're wasting your life. Everyone else is creating, building, showing up, and you're what? Lying around? Loser.

That word hit hard. And deep. I didn't even realize I was saying it to myself until it echoed in the silence one morning.

Being busy made me feel less like a loser.

I heard it like a confession in a church I hadn't entered in years.

When I produced, I felt like I had worth. When I had things to show, things to sell, things to post—I felt like I belonged. But now? With nothing on the timeline and no shiny thing to point to, I felt hollow, like a washed-up shell of a person who once mattered.

That morning, I sat with my tea and scrolled, watching everyone else out there doing things. Being inspiring. Making moves. Changing lives. And I felt small. Like I was disappearing. I closed the app. I sat with an ache in my chest. And then, almost instinctively, I stood up.

I walked to the speaker and pressed play. A beat came on, low and slow. Something with heat in it. With an *invitation*. I let my hips sway. My arms rise. My chest opened. And then I danced—not for exercise, not to be fixed, but because this was how I prayed. And as I moved, something happened.

I felt strong again. Alive. Lit from within. I could see her: the me I dreamed of being.

I could see the stage. The lights. My voice soaring through a mic, through a crowd, through time. I felt the music pouring from my body, not for approval, but because it was what I was born to do.

I wasn't chasing the dream. It *was* the dream. And in that moment, it wasn't some far-off fantasy.

It was *real*. It was *me*.

And yet, even as that vision rose, so did the grief, because I keep piling other things on top of it. Tasks. Projects. Responsibilities. All these half-finished things I convinced myself I "had" to do before I earned the right to do the thing I *actually* love.

I buried the dream under the to-do list. I numbed the voice with obligation. But my body remembered. When I dance, I remember who I am, what I came here to do, and that she's already in me—powerful, radiant, embodied. I just had to stop abandoning her. I had to stop choosing everything else first.

But the next day, I forgot again. The high wore off. The calendar called. The notifications piled up. Suddenly, I was deep in admin, booking, building, replying, and fixing.

Halfway through the day, I realized I hadn't moved. I hadn't sung. I hadn't danced. I went right back to filling space with work. That familiar loop came back.

You can't do that dream stuff until you finish this other stuff. Who do you think you are to prioritize joy right now? There's too much to do. There's always too much to do.

And I almost believed it. Again. Until I walked past the mirror and caught a glimpse of her—the woman from the dance. The one who sang like fire. The one who knew. And she just looked at me like:

Really? You're going to abandon me again?

I stopped. Took a breath. Closed the laptop. Stepped outside. Let the sun hit my face.

And I promised.

I'm trying. I really am.

This healing, this remembering, is not a linear process.

Sometimes I forget. Sometimes, I resist. However, I'm learning to respond more quickly.

To dance before the spiral swallows me. To sing before the doubt gets too loud. To choose myself in the little moments, not just the big declarations. Because the dream isn't waiting somewhere far away.

She's here—in my feet, in my lungs, in my voice. And she'll keep rising as long as I keep listening.

THE TOOL

DANCE AS DEVOTION

A Ritual for Remembering Who You Are

We live in a world that tells us rest must be earned, and dreams must be postponed. We're only valuable when we're producing, achieving, and performing. But your body knows a different truth.

When we move without an agenda, we return to something primal and holy. We shake loose the stories, the shame, the stuckness. We stop managing and start feeling.

This is the medicine that found me in my kitchen: Ecstatic dance, not as a performance, but as prayer.

Not as choreography but as *communion*.

So, if you're ready to meet yourself again—not in the mirror, but in motion—this ritual is for you.

Ecstatic Dance Ritual: A ten- to twenty-minute embodiment practice.

What You'll Need:

- A space where you can move freely (your bedroom, living room, backyard)
- A speaker or headphones
- A playlist with a beginning, build, climax, and release (see suggested structure below)
- Optional: journal, candle, essential oil, or dim lighting

1. Set the Space

Light a candle or place your hands over your heart.

Take a few deep breaths and whisper:

I am here to remember.

I do not have to earn this joy. I only have to allow it.

Release any expectations. This is not a performance.

2. Choose Your Music

Build your playlist like a wave:

- Opening track (gentle): Slow, ambient, grounded
- Build (two to three tracks): Mid-tempo, soulful, or sensual
- Climax (one to two tracks): Big, bold, emotional, primal
- Release (one track): Soft, melodic, integrating

Or search for "Ecstatic Dance / 5 Rhythms" playlist on Spotify or YouTube.

3. Begin to Move

Let your breath lead your body.

Let your feet root to the earth.

Let your hands tell the story.

There are no wrong movements. No wrong feelings.

If grief comes, let it.

If rage moves through, welcome it.

If joy erupts, give it space to rise.

Trust your body. It knows the way.

4. Close with Stillness

When the music fades, sit or lie down.

Place a hand on your chest, one on your belly.

Breathe.

Listen.

Feel.

Say aloud or write:

What did I feel?

What part of me came alive?

What am I remembering?

OPTIONAL JOURNAL PROMPTS:

Take a moment. Close your eyes. Breathe into your body.

- What am I suppressing that my body wants to express?
- What moves me toward joy, even in stillness?
- What does power feel like in my body today?
- What is the dream I keep burying under my to-do list?
- What parts of me come alive when no one's watching?
- Where do I feel most powerful, most honest, most *me*—and what would it take to choose that version of myself more often?
- What is my body asking for?
- What have I been postponing that my soul is ready to claim—*now?*

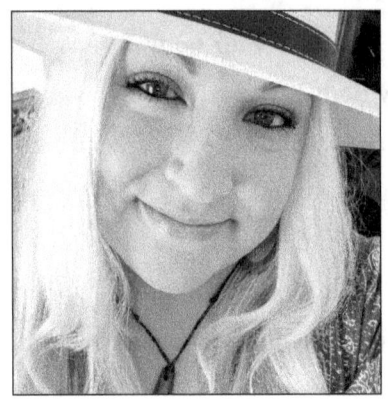

Dr. Tiffany McBride (she/her, they/them) is a Doctor of Shamanic Psycho-Spiritual Studies, a clinical licensed psychotherapist, a creative life coach, trauma recovery guide, an energy master and teacher, a birth and death doula, an ordained shamanic minister, an expressive musician and artist, and a four-time bestselling author. Tiffany runs a practice named Holistic Vibrations, LLC, utilizing integrative remedies and altered states of consciousness for those who struggle with trauma, addictions, women's issues, LGBTQAI+ support, and those seeking a deeper spiritual connection with their intuition.

After over 20 years of experience and work, Tiffany embodies the essence of an ultimate resource guide to holistic and clinical healing. They weave ancient wisdom with modern therapeutic techniques to guide others toward wholeness and self-discovery. Their path has been a relentless pursuit of knowledge, compassion, and service to humanity.

Looking towards the future, Tiffany envisions spreading their knowledge and medicine through online courses, classes, retreats, and workshops worldwide, empowering individuals to embark on their healing journeys. With their blend of clinical expertise, holistic healing, spiritual wisdom, and compassionate presence, Tiffany inspires and uplifts those they encounter, guiding them toward healing, transformation, and self-discovery.

Tiffany loves to write, make candles, create art, play the ukulele and guitar, sing, write music, dance, be in nature, take photographs, go to concerts, and connect with friends when she isn't working.

Connect with Tiffany:

Website: https://www.tiffany-mcbride.org
https://www.themysticmuse.org

Instagram: https://www.instagram.com/witchycrowwmn83

Facebook:
https://www.facebook.com/profile.php?id=61552573784401
https://www.facebook.com/profile.php?id=61576753293948

CHAPTER 16

Not for Their Approval

Creating Self-Love Through Creativity

Leah Johnson

MY STORY

Just once, I wanted them to see me. Not the gaslit moments, where they pretended to see me, but *see* me.

I don't know why—maybe because of trauma—but my brain is often short on specifics over time. I have a hard time recounting word for word all the mean, horrific, sexist, degrading, demoralizing, demeaning statements spewed at me over the years. Still, I will never forget how they made me feel.

It seems emotional memories are timeless. The feeling I was the dirt of the Earth, an unworthy mutant, a pawn in their game of power, a weak damsel who needed saving, a constant failure, not smart enough, not experienced enough, not accomplished enough to get the credibility I deserved—those feelings lived in my bones.

They took up residence in the pores of my being as a child—an invasive species, planted and then slowly overtook every part of my soul, whispering into my being the inadequacy of my existence over and over. "You're not enough. You will never be enough."

* * *

I walked into the backyard. White tents peaked the skyline backdrop of the Colorado mountains. People strolled the lawn, wearing as close to Hamptons summer attire as we get in my small town. I looked down at what I wore, woefully underdressed in my jean shorts and vibrant blue three-quarter sleeve cotton shirt. *At least I put on my favorite pair of earrings and a little makeup.*

My feral-looking children trailed me, like following Mama Duck. In all my years in local politics, this was a common place to find them. I arrived at events strewn with "prestigious" people, accompanied by the little ones in tow. I at least felt good about how far I always pushed this boundary in my time in politics. Before, I always arrived at these events with a motive: to work the room—or the backyard in this case—and find the person with the story, the connection, the information I might need to broker some political deal. I told myself my motives were driven by a visceral love for my community, to ensure it remained the great place I was fortunate to grow up in.

Although my intentions were always pure, I now realize how clear my motives were: I wanted to prove something to these people.

This time, walking into the event was different. I wasn't walking in with something to prove; I didn't care if I talked to anyone, except the person I was there to support. I freed myself from this life—broke up with it six months before. I walked away, quit it all, and said, "Enough." I moved my family to Mexico for three months, but that was just a quick exit strategy, and with no long-term plan—aren't we constantly working on that? I had to return to the place I still called home, even if it felt like a prison of my pain.

By quitting, I made a statement to myself, even if they didn't see it. Enough of the constant pursuit of success, the continuous striving to be seen, to be recognized, to be acknowledged, to honor just one accomplishment, to have them just once value my voice, my offerings, my existence. I was only here because it was a celebration of life, and my friend—one of the few in the whole thing—had lost his partner. Being there to support him was important.

That sense of duty led me straight into wounds that weren't even fully scabbed over yet, ripping delicate protection off in one quick motion. But the rawness led to a release I so desperately needed. As I moved further into the space, I became overtly aware of all the wounds that existed, like walking back into an abusive relationship or relapsing in addiction. My experience has encompassed and represented both. *This time, I'm not getting sucked in.*

And this time, while I felt a great deal of sadness, it was the closure I needed.

I felt like an observer, having an almost out-of-body experience.

My demeanor was reserved. I imagined myself blending into the background, not there in human form at all. I saw my wounds outside of me, hovering over specific individuals. The memories of the emotions they caused me were attached to them and what they represented, not to me. It was as if I looked out at a sea of memories, each floating over the grass, holding a plastic wine glass and dressed up in fancy attire. But these memories didn't sit inside me, as they had for all those years; what I soon came to realize is I was different now, and they couldn't take that away from me.

As I scanned the crowd, I realized over the years, I kissed the ring of so many of these people in the name of progress, which still made me a little nauseous. The characters spanned the political spectrum; it wasn't about politics, it was about money, power, and approval.

Approval was what I believed these people would give me, and with that, a louder voice and a platform to prove myself worthy. That would replace the pain with a sense of belonging—that sense of worthiness I so desperately desired.

Even if my wounds were ripped open by my mere presence amongst these people, there was something different about me now. I gained new awareness, self-love, a deeper sense of self-preservation, and a profound understanding of myself, all while honoring who I was by quitting.

I returned the pain to where it belonged, back into the space where I so fervently sought approval. It floated out of me, back into where it was birthed, and then set behind the mountains with the Colorado sun. It was a ceremony for the death of who I once was.

I sat amongst these people, sad and uncomfortable, but I felt a power like never before. Unlike all the times before when I got sucked back in—when they pandered to my desire to be seen—this time, all I wanted to do was run as fast as I could in the other direction. That feeling was even further confirmation that I was headed down the right path.

The people in that backyard represented so much of what I needed to let go of, and now I had given myself the chance to do that: walk in and walk out, still holding strong to my sense of self. For the first time in my life, I successfully did this.

We must grieve what was, as burying it will never make it go away.

I needed to enter this space one last time to confirm I was on the right track, even if I loathed every minute of the experience. You must look the pain straight in the eye and say, "You no longer serve me; I set you free." It's in the raw that life gets real, and if I'm willing, where I heal the most.

As we got in the car and drove away, I started crying—perhaps the first real cry I had about leaving that life behind in six months, or ever, because it was literally in the rear-view mirror. Sobbing, I held on to the steering wheel as my kids, alarmed, consoled me, asking, "Mommy, are you okay?"

I replied, "You know what? Yes, I'm okay. I'm just sad they could never see me for who I am, but that's okay, because I see myself for who I am, and I believe that at the end of the day, that counts more than anything. And I want you two beautiful little beings to know, you never need anyone's approval from the outside. What matters most is you love yourselves from the inside out, and Mommy loves you from the outside all the way deep into those amazing little hearts of yours."

The emotion in the car was a grief that needed to happen—for me, for the idea that sat within me so long, for the feelings of unworthiness, and for the fact that those people were never going to give me that sense of worth I sought, ever.

I grieved and celebrated all at once because in that rawness, in the uncomfortable, is where actual change and breakthroughs happen. I recognized the pain was no longer something to hold in my being or my soul, and there was so much more yet to come in my unfolding. I was done with that life, and it felt so good!

* * *

To understand how I arrived at the moment when I released my desperate need for external approval, we must go back to my childhood.

My mom in human form wasn't great. Over the last 12 years, I've built an entirely different relationship with her in spirit form, but the wounds of her time on Earth remain, even after all the work I've done. The longing I had for approval from all the blue bloods of my town was the same longing I had for my mother: just to be seen and honored for who I was and what I had to offer. After her death, the need for approval just transferred to a larger pool, which would never quench that thirst.

At its core, my seeking approval was rooted in my mother. I was an honor student, student body president, captain of the debate team, and captain of the golf team (both in high school and college). I earned a golf scholarship to a prestigious university and had a successful national political career. None of it was good enough to make me feel seen. None of it was worthy of three simple words every child longs to hear from their mother: I love you.

She died, and 12 years later, I ended up in a backyard, finally understanding, for the first time in my life, deep down in my cells in every part of my being, I was never going to get the approval I sought from the collective of those people. And it wasn't coming from my mom, either. The realization was crushing and freeing all at once.

While my mom is gone and her whispers in the spirit of "I love you" are plentiful these days, it's simply not the same as savoring a moment where you remember love physically around you, touching your skin, smelling the intention, hearing the compassion, and seeing a softness. There were no warm blankets of memories to wrap around me, reminding me I was loved. And I certainly wasn't going to get it from a time and place in the local political world; that was simply the delusion that success and accomplishments would fill that void and finally make me seen for the vibrant, intelligent, compassionate, and dedicated person I am.

But none of that was coming.

It was like a scene in a movie where the main character sits, waiting for the love of their life to arrive at a candlelit dinner.

The waiter keeps checking in, and the person keeps checking their watch: "He'll be here. I know it." But he never arrives.

What I finally realized is the love of my life was already here: it was me. No one was going to give me the validation or love I sought. I had to give it to myself.

I was the one I had been waiting for. I was the love and approval that had been there all along. I just had to be brave enough to see it, brave enough to believe it, and brave enough to stop seeking it in places I was never going to find it.

And so, I sought *my* approval and quit politics to become a painter. I left the rat race and now lead retreats for women to Teotihuacán, Mexico, as well as Intentional Creativity® Workshops, all designed to empower women to delve deeper into themselves, their creativity, and their souls, ultimately helping them understand the divine within. You don't need approval from the outside; the love you have for yourself in your heart is enough, because we're all enough just as we are.

I quit the desperate need for approval and found a peace I didn't even know was possible. I stopped people-pleasing and started Leah-pleasing. My nervous system is so thankful.

I speak, I write, I paint, I create, and I live with intentional joy and gratitude. If you asked me at the climax of my life in politics if such a life was possible, I would have laughed you off. My denial wouldn't let my soul hear the truth—but no more.

No more gaslighting, no more lack of gratitude, no more watching twice the money go to others for sub ideas and experiences to mine. No more saying the same things over and over, only for them to have value when a white man says them. No more emotional and mental abuse, no more doubting myself. No more seeking my worthiness in them.

My life journey taught me I am enough. My life is not for their approval; my approval is all I need.

THE TOOL

Creativity has always been my outlet for healing, allowing me to enter a state of flow and realize the power and wisdom within me all along. Long before I had the words to describe what I was doing, I journaled with color, cuttings from magazines, writings, poetry, and words, photos, stickers—anything that could stick to a page in a book that honored who I was, the pain I harbored, and my longing for hope and joy.

When I became trained as an Intentional Creativity® instructor and began to put clear words to the actions I took for years, it became clear to me: The power to heal ourselves is within each of us. We're created to heal; that's how our souls evolve into the highest versions of ourselves.

For me, more than any other way, the power of healing is rooted deeply in my ability to create. My ability to shift my energy from one of pain to joy through a pen, marker, or paintbrush ignited my life, my energy, and my power of self-love more than any other healing activity I invested my time in.

"I AM LOVED" JOURNAL

Materials:

- Several sheets of paper
- Yarn and a hole punch
- Old magazines
- Markers, colored pencils, acrylic markers (some coloring devices)
- Optional: stickers, glitter, dried flowers—anything you can put on a page that calls to you

Step 1: Take the few sheets and fold them in half. Along the crease line, poke some holes so you can sew yarn through the fold crease, creating a small book.

Step 2: Create a cover that conveys this is a self-love journal.

Step 3: Start anywhere in the book; it doesn't have to be on the first page. Create love letters, love poems, love pictures, or designs. Focus on your strengths and callings that come from deep within you, not the external voices. Perhaps pick this up after your meditation, shamanic journey, or your practice to connect to your higher power. When we're open spiritually and then allow ourselves to activate our creativity, the power of reawakening our wisdom is something fierce.

Each thing you add to the journal should be done with intention—something you love about yourself, something you're grateful for about yourself—a celebration and an act of honoring, releasing the need for approval, and revealing just how amazing you are. Use the journal as a tool to return to over and over again, turning pages and words, layers and colors into a testament of how amazing you are as a human.

To see photos and a fun video of an example of an *"I Am Loved"* *Journal*, visit www.findingfantasticjoy.com/hch.

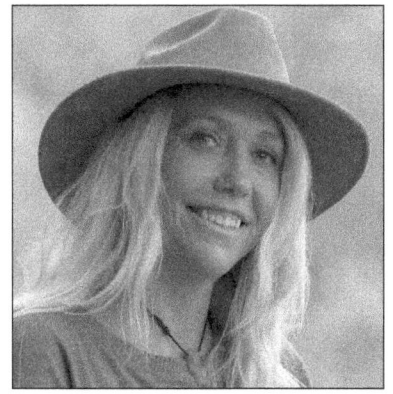

Leah Johnson is a former elected official-turned artist, author, and transformational guide who helps people reconnect with their creativity, reclaim their joy, and live more intentionally. After a 25-year career in politics and public affairs, including roles with national campaigns and as a city councilwoman, Leah experienced a silent breakdown beneath the weight of burnout, perfectionism, and the pressure to achieve. What looked successful on the outside felt increasingly hollow within.

Her path to healing began not with policy, but with a paintbrush. Through intentional creativity and spiritual inquiry, Leah began to peel back the layers of who she was told to be—and rediscovered the vibrant, creative soul she always was. That transformation became the foundation for her life's new work: helping others shed roles, expectations, and old stories to reconnect with their joy and create lives they want to live.

Today, Leah is the founder of Finding Fantastic Joy and leads immersive retreats in sacred spaces, such as Teotihuacán, Mexico, where women gather for deep, creative healing and ceremony. She's a certified Intentional Creativity® Teacher and Cura Guide, and the best-selling author of *Finding Fantastic Joy: How Building a Self-Advocacy Campaign Led Me Out of Darkness*. Her forthcoming book, *Girl! Baptize Yourself* invites women to spiritually and creatively reclaim their truth.

Through retreats, workshops, keynotes, and her art, Leah creates spaces where healing meets joy, where creativity becomes a sacred tool for transformation, and where each person is reminded: *You are the artist of your life—and your canvas is ready.*

She lives in Colorado with her family and believes joy is not a luxury—it's a lifeline.

Connect with Leah:

www.findingfantasticjoy.com

CHAPTER 17

The Hippie and the Old Rancher

Finding Freedom from Hatred Where Opposites Intersect

Nancy Terry

If we can stay with the tension of the opposites long enough...
sustain it, be true to it—we can sometimes become vessels
within which the divine opposites come together
and give birth to a new reality.

~ Marie Louise Von Franz

MY STORY

The marshal glanced absently at me as I sat quietly on a cold metal chair in a small office somewhere in the bowels of the federal courthouse. He snapped the handcuffs on first, then the leg irons. I remember looking at my husband, standing there in his nice, pressed dark suit, fresh out of the courtroom, a convicted felon now and forever.

"Hand her your keys and your watch and tell her goodbye." The marshal's voice was as flat and unemotional as I felt inside.

I watched two guards escort my children's father through the doorway and heard the chains clanging as he shuffled down the hall.

I don't remember the two-hour drive to my parents' house to pick up my kids. I don't remember much of anything except a dull, aching defeat.

I've done it again. Fucked up. Embarrassed the family. Let myself down…again.

Reluctantly, I made my way into their house and held tight to my kids while my mom cried, and my dad dismissively popped open another Budweiser. I didn't expect any emotional support from them, but then Dad surprised me. In a voice somewhat gentler than his usual tone, he offered this:

"You have two kids to raise. You have a chance to pull yourself up by your bootstraps, be strong, and turn your life around. Now get busy!"

I gathered up my baby boy and my five-year-old daughter, went home, and pulled up my bootstraps. While my mind screamed, "This is the worst day of your life!" my frozen heart melted, and the shackles of an unholy relationship turned to dust in the wind.

His incarceration day was my liberation day. The toxic masculinity I was immersed in from day one shaped my ideas about men and sent me on a crusade to save and fix the walking wounded.

If I just love them enough—if they just love me enough…

My dad, two older brothers, uncles, and male cousins were "men's men," and that involved drinking, fighting, shooting guns, and shamelessly ordering women around. They were hardworking, hard-drinking men who lived on the edge of anger.

Boys don't have emotions, only sissies do. They possessed some admirable qualities, too, but I hadn't yet mastered the art of compassion that justified their behaviors. I observed my mother and her sisters in unfulfilled marriages, complaining behind their husbands' backs, and wondered if there was another way. That was the late 60s, and veering off the expected path was easy. An energy deep inside invited me to walk away from the familiar and step into the unknown.

The problem was, I didn't have a roadmap, so I got lost a few more times.

THE HIPPIE

My sacred unraveling started during the summer between my junior and senior years of high school. Our carefree days were filled with flowers in our hair, bell-bottoms swaying to the music of The Mamas and the Papas, California dreaming, pot smoke rising, news of Woodstock, and voices calling for peace.

The shock of Kent State clouded my 16th birthday, and it became real for me that not everyone loved our summer of love. That included my parents, who had no idea what to do with me.

Psychedelics were our flashlights illuminating the outer world's turbulent chaos—and the inner world's, as well. After high school graduation, my girlfriends and I took off in our VW bus to look for America. We were empty and aching, and we didn't know why.

After the long, slow drive to Los Angeles and an initiation into big city life, we returned to the Midwest, rented a group of old farmhouses, and created a kind of communal living situation. We rejected materialism, including comforts like indoor plumbing and electricity. Free love, rock concerts, growing our food, chopping wood for heat, and lots of drugs sustained us for a while.

Then a bitterly cold winter froze our fantasies, and I was sick, cold, and hungry.

Maybe it's time to rethink my lifestyle.

There was tension in the opposites of my former and current life. Finding balance meant breathing life into the unlovable, shadow parts of myself I previously rejected.

As I look back at that young woman over 50 years ago, I'm inspired by her ability to find her way into and out of trouble, and to maintain deep, lifelong friendships, a zest for living, and a wicked sense of humor.

I not only love her, but I also really like her. A lot.

THE OLD RANCHER

When I asked the old rancher to tell me something he loved about ranch life, he said, "There's nothin' like building a straight mile of fence, lookin' back and feelin' proud."

I got it. Hard work. Blood, sweat, and tears, and the reward of pride for a job well done. Greg and I decided to weave our stories together to offer an authentic example of how two people with opposing views and ideals became a mirror for each other. We were both searching to restore balance to the divine feminine and masculine energies within us.

Greg's life and challenges could fill pages. Ranch life is hard work in all conditions and weather; then add to the mix a vindictive, alcohol-soaked father, always criticizing and demanding more. Greg had two brothers and a younger sister. His emotionally absent mother focused on the younger sister, who was a distraction from shattered dreams and the occasional black eye. That left the boys under the scrutiny of a wounded beast, who pitted them against each other in bloodbaths for his sick entertainment.

"What was it like, Greg, when your father watched you boys fight?" I asked him.

"I hated him. I was scared and knew I couldn't show it, or he would smell weakness, and I would be his next target," Greg responded. "In his sick mind, he was teaching us to be men. I learned to repress all my emotions to stay safe. Then one day, I had my fill with him. I was 12 years old, and he took me for a haircut. I refused to get my hair cut the way he wanted and embarrassed him in front of the barber."

Greg paused, then finished. "I knew I was in for a beating later, but decided right then, this son of a bitch is not going to win."

Injuries from work, fights, and sports piled up. Pain became a constant companion throughout Greg's life, starting with a shattered elbow at age four. That fall from a horse was the beginning of countless broken bones, concussions, sprains, and surgeries. He lived in a damaged body and described altercations and violence as routine. In his words:

When I look back, I often experienced what many call
'being in the zone.' It's that state of clear focus, strength, and
power that feels bigger than you. I've felt it during fights—not
because I wanted violence, but because I needed to defend
others. Most of the fights I was involved in were about standing
up for someone else. I learned early on that no one really wins a
fight, and that taught me something about myself.

I remember in seventh grade, I got in a fight with the school
bully. We went into the yard, and I hit him once.
He ended up with a headache, and I broke two knuckles,
which kept me in a cast for six weeks. I think we both learned
an important lesson that day.

Another time when I was outnumbered, I entered the 'zone'
and everything slowed down. I moved with strength and agility
that felt unreal. I don't think they touched me. I experienced
a clarity I can't explain. Maybe it was a spiritual awakening
beginning to stir, and access to a power that guides and protects.

Experiencing violence and conflict ironically set me on a path
of healing and self-discovery. Working with psychedelics and
other mind-expanding modalities opened my heart and gave
me peace. I'm grateful for how far I've come.

Before his indoctrination into the world of psychedelics, Greg received another message from an oracle, which he recognized as an affirmation.

He was working on his ranch one day, feeling alone and empty. While chopping down cedar saplings, he hit the base of one with his axe.

Whack!

He fell back as it exploded with ladybugs. Millions of ladybugs poured out of the tiny sapling and covered his clothes, the ground around him, and filled the sky above him. Life force energy was everywhere!

"What do you think it meant?" I asked him.

"It was a sign," he answered. "I was in awe and just sat there and watched this spectacle of nature, reassuring me all is well, and my purpose for this lifetime is being fulfilled. I felt peace and assurance moving forward. My past is teaching me acceptance and gratitude for the man I'm becoming."

My husband gently and openly introduced Greg to the expansive world of psychedelics to support his already growing curiosity. I quietly worked with people as a guide and offered microdosing for depression, anxiety, and other issues, as well as deeper journeys for healing and inspiration.

I was happy to share what I learned about the therapeutic use of plant medicines, even though Greg was not the typical inquirer. He was also the male stereotype I spent my life running from—and running into.

Something shifted in me as our work together evolved. He was new to the idea of self-discovery through inner journeys, but something ancient settled in his heart, and he fearlessly moved into unknown realms with ease, almost like he had been there before. During one session, Greg described the energy he saw.

"It's all around you, moving through your body and connecting with me. The colors from my hands are flowing into you, yours into mine. It's incredible! The blues, reds, greens, yellows are vibrant and alive!" He was ecstatic in his description.

The medicine taught him we're all interconnected, vibrational patterns. There is no "us and them." We're all living, breathing energy with endless possibilities of expression. That included his chronic pain, and he finally saw it as the great teacher of this lifetime. Sacred mushrooms opened doorways, and Greg stepped through them into new relationships with himself, his past, and the survival skills he outgrew long ago. The structure of a frightened, abused little boy built to protect against the big, bad world crumbled. I bore witness to a rebirth.

Greg's steady, consistent work continued for several years while his physical struggles lessened, layers of grief and anger fell away, and hope returned. Microdosing played an integral role in this success, alongside a gentle exercise program, a brilliant and innovative therapist, and a loving and supportive wife.

Greg called one day last summer.

"Hey! Guess what?! We're driving to Colorado in August, and I'm going to climb Mt. Handies! Fourteen thousand feet!"

I held the phone away from my ear. "Are you out of your mind?!"

"That's what my wife said, but if I'm going to help others who suffer with chronic pain, I need credibility. I'm doing it to prove to myself, too, that this psychedelic thing works!"

I chuckled and answered, "You know it works because you made it work! You couldn't walk 20 steps a couple of years ago. Your spine is still shaped like the letter *s*. What if you mess it all up?"

"Not going to. I'm training now. I'm going to do this or die trying. No worries, I'll be in the 'zone.'" He sounded resolute.

"Okay, you stubborn ol' rancher. I believe you, and you have my support."

And climb the fourteener, he did!

Greg said it was the hardest thing he has ever done, but his old back held out. It was breathing at that altitude that almost killed him. Standing at the top of Handies Peak was not only a physical feat of strength and determination, but a metaphorical achievement of bringing the past and present into alignment and birthing something new.

THE PAIN OF CONTRACTION VERSUS THE FREEDOM OF EXPANSION

So, how did all of this affect the little hippie girl? Her spirit will always live in my heart, and she'll always want to save the world. Witnessing Greg's transformation healed a part of me. He is, of course, still the old rancher who will defend and protect, but his heart has also made room for more compassion and acceptance.

And I'm finally able to make peace with the wounded masculine in my psyche, to suspend old programs, and to access a broader vision and clearer path to understanding.

Now I'm aware when I'm holding two opposing thoughts. The tension tells me to look deeper when feeling judgment, resistance, and separation.

What a long, strange trip it's been.

THE TOOL

I recently discovered a new visual practice that proved to be profound yet simple, and it brought much of what I've shared with you in this chapter into alignment.

Kintsugi, or golden joinery, is the Japanese art of mending broken pottery with gold lacquer without disguising the breakage, but instead retaining it as part of the history of the object. At the heart of kintsugi is wabi-sabi, or the practice of embracing imperfections and impermanence.

I never considered myself much of an artist, but years ago, my friend Emilie Collins taught me about elevating my deep inner wisdom and allowing my soul to teach me through art. I didn't need to have any artistic ability or training, either! Together, we created collages or painted with no intention of making a pretty picture.

And over time, the intuitive process has become one of my favorite ways to meditate. If we listen closely enough, we will hear our truth.

Kintsugi is the perfect metaphor for bringing the broken pieces back home. Gold is what gives us texture and color and illuminates us from within. Instead of repairing broken pottery, however, we can repair our broken selves using simple supplies:

- Gold paint
- Paintbrushes
- Paper or card stock
- Glue stick
- Images and photos

Allow the graphics to choose you as you look through magazine images and old photographs. The image may be a photo of you or something that represents an aspect of you, such as power, anger, love, or stubbornness. There may be a picture or graphic that reminds you of a role you are currently playing or have played in the past, such as mother, father, spouse, professional, sibling, or friend. It might be an image of a house that represents you or a place in nature that inspires you.

Mainly, trust that what shows up is what your inner healer is ready to work with.

If nothing definite strikes you, choose several images, and as you move into the process, you will know.

We will not tear up or destroy the images in any way. That language carries negative energy. The purpose and value of this exercise is to rework something within by disassembling and reassembling it in a way that represents the beauty of our imperfections and broken places.

For my recent experience, I chose a picture of myself from when I was 17, just beginning my rebellious years. I also chose a picture of myself from when I was 3 years old, all dressed up for the photographer to capture my innocence.

I didn't tear the photographs but instead placed them side by side, allowing both the innocent one and the tormented one to coexist. I surrounded them with gold paint, and both were perfect at that moment.

The 17-year-old, who carried a great deal of shame and confusion, found the gold paint to be a healing balm. And the little girl remembered how to shine! Everything would work out perfectly.

Journaling or writing about your creation later adds another layer of awareness to the messages that emerge. A simple 10-minute writing using a prompt like, "If I ask the gold paint to speak, it would tell me...," or, "When I tore the family photo, I remembered a time when..."

The kintsugi experience, along with writing this chapter, has unearthed long-buried memories that have been transformed from trauma to treasure. I'm grateful for Greg, who trusted me with his story and was as much my teacher as I was his.

I'm grateful for the people on this life path who believed in me until I was ready to take the reins and ride.

I'm grateful to Emilie, who helped me discover my inner artist! For more information about intuitive art opportunities, check out her website below.

I'm grateful for the Monday night women's group, which has been going strong for five years! It has become the cauldron where we play, learn, and share, with Patty being the rudder that steers our boat. I hope you, too, are in community with people you love.

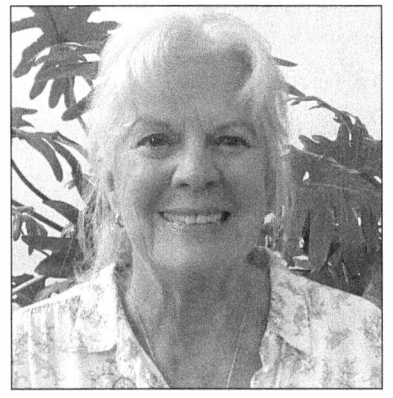

Nancy Terry is a retired social worker with over 30 years of experience as a certified sign language interpreter. Her years working with the Deaf community were deeply meaningful, and she took great pleasure in being a voice advocating for access and inclusion. Her deaf friends taught her so much about patience and acceptance.

After retiring from social work, Nancy became a certified family law mediator, once again stepping into the role of supporting those whose voices are often overlooked.

Many years ago, after an extended stay in the Peruvian jungles, she was reminded of the profound healing potential found in sacred plant medicines and ceremonial work. She studied with San Pedro shamans, ayahuascaros, and curanderos, and this experience reignited her lifelong passion for non-ordinary states of consciousness and the transformative powers they offer.

Nancy currently co-facilitates retreats at Half Moon Ranch in Castlerock, Colorado. The retreats offer sacred medicine journeys, integrative workshops, sound baths, yoga, breathwork, and energetic healing with horses.

Nancy lives in Northern Colorado with her husband and their cat, Hank.

For info on upcoming retreats:

Website: https://halfmoonranchretreats.com

Connect with Emilie Collins and find *your* inner artist:

Website: https://artbreathsoul.com

Want more info or just want to chat:

Email: nancy@addisonterry.com

CHAPTER 18

The Question That Freed Me

How to Heal Anything

R. Scott Holmes

MY STORY

All my life, I've worked so hard at being a friend. Where is everybody?

James Taylor's "You've Got a Friend" plays softly in the background as I sit in the well-worn, overstuffed recliner, absentmindedly scratching behind the cat's ears.

How many hours have I been sitting here? How does time just escape me now?

This house used to be so full of life with kids, animals, and to-do lists. And now I have to remind myself to get out of bed.

Carole King's "So Far Away" plays, and it seems I can't feel or touch the life I once had.

The songs playing on the radio understand, as if they're performing just for me. It feels like finding love as a 13-year-old, when all those silly love songs finally make sense.

Where did I go, and why am I so far away?

That was nine years ago, just after my wife of 39 years succumbed to her 20-year breast cancer battle. She was a warrior until she became a patient. The constant beatings from treatments left her a brittle shell, trying not to crack under the weight of survival.

So, you're asking yourself, "What's the question?"

I sat at the wooden bar at a reception, speaking with Lees, a lithe and limber coworker. We started talking about yoga. She practiced since college and was a high-level instructor. Being a smart-ass 50-year-old know-it-all, I said, "That's for women who have nothing better to do."

"Oh, really? Bend over and touch your toes, right now!"

I slid smoothly from the barstool, bent over, and reached all the way to my knees. I couldn't move any further, no matter how I strained.

"I guess I'm just a stiff white guy," I said, embarrassed at my performance.

"I'll see you Saturday at nine at the health club," she said as she peacocked away.

Is this something I'm really going to do?

It felt right. I was out of shape, had no flexibility, and was stuck in my routine of no routine. I showed up with my newly bought discount store yoga mat, not knowing what to expect.

Twenty women side-eyed me as I walked to the very back corner of the room, hoping not to be noticed. The lights darkened, and meditation music started. Lees gave succinct instructions on positions, allowing variations for those who couldn't quite complete the pose.

After an hour of sweating, grunting, and hurting in places I didn't know were even a part of my body, Lees asked how I liked it.

"Not bad. I might even show up next week," I answered. She smiled and gave my arm a reassuring squeeze.

I did show up the next week, and I started practicing the poses at home in between classes. My back, which put me out of commission for a week at a time, felt amazing. I didn't feel 70 years old when I got out of bed. My knees, which bothered me since my teenage years, didn't ache anymore. I stood taller and straighter than ever before.

Yoga really is the answer to the question of my aging body. I'm glad I said yes.

I went to yoga for five years every week without fail. Years later, it's now a daily part of my practice, even though I don't go to classes very often. And I can still touch my toes.

So, you're asking yourself, "What's the question?"

A friend, Patti, suggested going to a young medium she met. My wife Moira had been gone nearly a year, and even though I didn't understand or know if I believed in the practice, I went out of curiosity. *It'll be good for a laugh.*

Patti went into the room first for about 40 minutes and came out clutching Kleenex with tears streaming down her face. She lost her mom recently and was desperate to connect.

"Come in," said Samantha, a 20-something beauty with a bright smile. "The Kleenex is right beside you."

"Don't worry, I'm not a crier. I won't need them."

Samantha proceeded to describe Moira as she looked when she was 30 to a T.

"Moira wants you to know she's sorry. She couldn't recover after the loss of your daughter. She says she never said thank you enough, and there was no one else she would rather go into battle with than you."

Tears cascaded down my face. I couldn't catch them all. This was one of the few times my wife had apologized to me, and it was from the great beyond!

"Moira is with your daughter. They no longer feel the pains they experienced here on Earth."

I suddenly felt lighter as the weight of losing my daughter and wife slid slowly from my shoulders. They were at peace, and maybe I could find that peace within me.

The answer to my grief is in front of me. So glad I said yes to this session. It changes my perspective on everything.

I continued sessions with Samantha through the years, with amazing revelations and results.

So, you're asking yourself, "What's the question?"

I strained to hear Paul in the noisy café as we reminisced about our plans to travel after college. I settled down and had a family while Paul traveled the globe, started multiple businesses, and then found life with children was what he needed.

"Why don't we recreate the adventure we always talked about? Europe, but not as poor students." We were both just turning 60.

I was unencumbered with caregiving for the first time in 35 years, and the chance to finally see Europe after all these years called to me.

Am I being selfish in taking this trip? Could I? Should I?

Disembarking from the Iberia Airline jet in Munich had me pinching myself. The 17-day driving journey was about to start. We settled into a black Audi Q7 diesel SUV for the ride of our lives: 2500 miles and infinite memories.

We traveled through Munich, Nuremberg, Furth, Dresden, and Mannheim, Germany; Prague, Czech Republic; Strasbourg, France: Basel, Geneva, Lausanne, Lucerne, and Zurich, Switzerland; Lake Cuomo and Venice, Italy; Ljubljana, Slovenia; Bratislava, Slovakia; Vienna, Linz, and Salzburg, Austria. We returned to Munich in time for Oktoberfest.

"Hey Paul, tomorrow is my 60th birthday. Let's do something extra special."

Paul planned the epic day. Breakfast in Germany. Lunch in France. Dinner in Switzerland.

Here I am, celebrating with my best friend in Europe. I never believed this was possible, yet here I am.

So, you're asking yourself, "What's the question?"

A teacher of mine suggested I look into this publishing house that was doing collaborations with writers who focus on different modalities. I contacted Laura Di Franco, and she suggested I become an advanced reader for a compilation that was coming out. I could review the book before publication.

I'm just starting my energy journey and don't know my ass from a hole in the ground. How could anything I have to say be of value to anyone?

Laura emailed me and asked if she could put the review on the back cover of the book.

Are you kidding me? That is the most exciting thing in my very short wannabe-writing career.

Trying to sound as professional as possible, I told her that if she would like to use the quote, I wouldn't mind. I was out-of-my-mind ecstatic. *Wow, my words are being seen!*

Two weeks later, Laura called and said I should speak to a lead author about a book she was putting together. I contacted Hemali Vora, and we talked about grief, loss, and what they mean. I was honored to be asked to contribute, but how could I write 3000 words on my story? I could barely share it with another living soul without breaking down.

Moira, the lifelong teacher, would ask me to share her story so others can learn and find comfort in those words. I'll do this to honor her.

It took me 30 sleepless days and nights to put my story into words. The right words. Grappling with all the emotions exhumed the loss of my daughter and wife. Tear-stained legal pads were the vehicle that transported my grief, happiness, sadness, and joy into being.

Is it good enough? What will my family say? Will anyone read this or even care about it?

Three revisions and numerous "Can you read this and tell me what you think?" requests later, with fear bursting out at the seams, "Your Path is Revealed: Transforming from Caregiving to Self-Caring" in *Sacred Death: 25 Tools for Caregivers* was born. It's an Amazon bestseller for Brave Healer Publications.

This was a turning point in my life after dealing with the losses of my 15-year-old daughter, my 60-year-old wife, my lifelong identity, and the heaviness of grief that permeated every pore, every cell, every day.

So, you're asking yourself, "What's the question?"

Indian meditation music played in the small office where Samantha, the medium, worked. Small statues, incense wafting throughout the tight space, brightly colored wall hangings, and cozy pillows made the space warm and welcoming.

"It's good seeing you again. Please sit, and we'll start the reading."

I don't know what I'm expecting. After these last few years, I need some direction—if I even have a direction.

As the reading started, Sam looked to her right and started having a conversation with someone I couldn't see.

"No, I don't understand. What is Penang? Tell him what? He has to what? Wait, I don't understand!"

I sat in rapt attention, wondering what just happened.

"The gentleman is one of your guides—older, long white beard, and very short on explanation. He said you're to go to the Burmese Hindu Temple in Penang to collect your soul parts. And I'm not sure what any of that means."

Well, if she didn't understand that, how the hell was I supposed to make sense of it?

We looked up Penang, an island off the coast of Malaysia. We looked up the Dhammikarama Burmese Temple, and sure enough, there was only one, with a 40-foot-tall, golden-robed Buddha. Collecting soul parts was something she'd heard about from a shaman, but she wasn't sure what the practice involved.

"What am I supposed to do about this?" I asked.

"This is about you and your guides; I'm just the messenger."

Paul and I were heading on a 17-day guided tour of Thailand, Cambodia, and Vietnam the next month. How was I supposed to get to Malaysia?

The experiences in Bangkok, Phnom Penh, Ho Chi Min City, Hoi An, Hanoi, and Ha Long Bay were otherworldly. There were times when, even though I had never been to Southeast Asia, I felt at home. I couldn't shake the feeling that I had come here before.

One month after getting back from our whirlwind trip, I received an email from the tour company we used. There was a tour of Singapore and Malaysia on the list. I opened the email and looked through the itinerary. Sure enough, the last destination was Penang, and the hotel was three blocks from the Burmese Temple.

How will I pull this off? Do I really want to travel halfway around the world on the word of someone I can't see and a medium who has no clue what to do?

"How would you like to take a trip that will take 24 hours on a plane?" I asked. "You won't know the language, may not like the food, you'll be on a bus with 30 other people, and it's going to be hot."

Patti paused for five seconds and said, "Sure, I'll go anywhere in the world with you."

Shaun, our tour guide in Malaysia, was five feet of energy, knowledge, and good humor. I explained why we were on the tour and that on the last day, I would make a pilgrimage to the Burmese Temple in our free time.

The tour was stunning, showing the best of Malay culture, historic sites, and history. On the last day of the tour, Shaun announced, "We have an extra special stop. This is the Dhammikarama Burmese Temple where you'll see the reclining Buddha and the majestic, 40-foot standing Buddha." He winked to let me know it was his gift to me.

The spotless marble floor in the open-air temple felt cool as I slowly walked toward the statue. Stunning in gold robes, the marble statue seemed to glow. Gold filigree symbols painted the walls.

What am I supposed to do now? I traveled thousands of miles to be here, and I don't understand any of this. If I just listen and feel into it, maybe something will come to me.

Slowly, I opened myself up to possibility. "Those lost soul parts—if they're meant for me, I invite them to come home." In my mind's eye, three orbs of light descended from behind the Buddha and glided down through my crown chakra.

I heard, "Welcome home," and my heart felt like it would burst. I stood, transfixed, until a tap on my shoulder brought me back.

"We have to go; the bus is waiting." Slowly, I walked back with Patti arm-in-arm; we were the last ones on the bus.

So, you're asking yourself, "What's the question?"

The whip-poor-will's sharp voice and Bradford Tilden's thrumming sound bowl reverberated throughout the room. Forty people sat transfixed as the vibrations made their cells sing. This was just the beginning of a five-day retreat in upstate New York.

Laura Di Franco had brought together a band of healers, artists, and business mavens in the ultimate collaboration of fun, business, and magic.

Blindfolded, lying on mats, and covered in Peruvian blankets, I was transported to my past, my future, and so many versions of myself during a breathwork experience produced by Jeremy Pager and Stephanie Urbina Jones. The music physically moved me in a kaleidoscope of images and sensations.

"Thank you so much for that experience; it was once in a lifetime," I said to Jeremy.

He replied, "If you think that was amazing, you should come with us to Peru. Machu Picchu is great, but it's not the highlight."

Having Machu Picchu on my bucket list raised my curiosity.

Am I ready for a shamanic journey? Am I in a place to transform this experience?

Five months later, I landed in Cusco, Peru, after 15 hours of travel. Jorge Luis Delgado was our guide, shaman, and host. We visited Incan sites too numerous to mention, as every turn on the winding roads revealed new vistas and awe-inspiring architecture. At each stop, we performed rituals and felt into the vibration and energy.

Jorge instructed us at the Condor Temple: "Pour this mixture into the ground. Ask Pacha Mama to accept this gift. Form a triangle with your thumbs and forefingers. At your base chakra, invite the golden serpent of creation in. Allow it all the way up through your crown. When you're done, place your hands on the Condor rock to take any dark or unwanted energy."

The second I placed my hands on the rock, torrents of grief, sadness, and pain poured through me. I sobbed uncontrollably.

Where is all this sorrow coming from? This can't be all mine. Why can't I stop heaving, trying to catch my breath? I've never felt emotions sweep over me like windswept waves pounding the beach, unrelenting.

When I finally caught my breath, I turned from the rock only to be embraced by two of our traveling family. They didn't say a word, just held me in their hug until I could stand on my own.

I believe I released generations of pain and anguish from my family. My hope is they can accept the gift.

So, you're asking yourself, "What's the question?"

THE TOOL

Sit comfortably, eyes closed, and remember a time when you were eight or 11 or 14 or 17 years old. Feel into the joy of being a kid and exploring the world around you. Put on some of the music you loved at that time—you know, the one that brings that "yeah, baby" feeling.

Everything was possible. Your whole life was before you, and your curious, adventurous spirit dictated what excited and intrigued you. Everything was new. Feel it completely.

Open your eyes, and you're 42 or 55 or 67. You've lived quite a bit of life. You've had great and not-so-great experiences. Loved and lost more than you care to remember. So many responsibilities. So little time.

What is the question, you ask?

Is this for me?

Do you hear that small voice? The one you heard as your younger self?

Do you remember how that voice guided you before it was replaced by the voices of your parents, your girlfriend, your husband, your boss, or your family?

Wait. How does that heal anything I'm feeling right now?

Your 18-year-old soul still resides within you, and it's looking forward to what the rest of your life has to offer. When you clear all the layers that have been smothered, changed, and twisted through years of living, there it is:

Your authentic self!

The one you used to know. Finding that part within is how you heal the pain, the confusion, the discomfort you're living with right now.

The answer is finding you, no matter the journey or modality. You.

Clarity awaits in listening to that voice. It never left you. Quietly asking the question will give you the whispered response you need to hear.

The rest of your life is waiting. Live it joyfully, skipping, laughing, and smiling that shit-eating grin only your best friend understands.

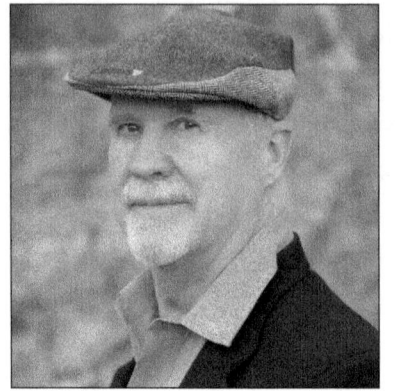

R. Scott Holmes is an intuitive energy practitioner and transformational coach using Reiki, Polarity Therapy, RYSE, ThetaHealing, and Find Your Voice coaching techniques to clear, ground, and align your energetic body. His specialty is collaborating with professional men and women, allowing them to heal and maintain their true paths in life.

He began walking in the holistic healing world when his wife of 39 years died after a 20-year battle with breast cancer. After years of caregiving for his daughter and wife, the world of coaching, healing, and energy opened. His soul journey has been to help heal others through one-on-one sessions, teaching, and volunteering.

Walk with him to find the rituals and daily practices enabling you to open those locked spaces. Allow your most authentic self to shine through and embrace the life you are living.

Contact Scott for a free thirty-minute share to see if you can unwrap the questions carried in your heart.

Connect with Scott:

Website: https//www.rscottholmes.com

Email: rscott_holmes@yahoo.com

Facebook: https//www.facebook.com/Scott.Holmes.31105674

Instagram: https//www.instagram.com/r.scottholmes

CHAPTER 19

The Frequency Within

A Journey of Self-Attunement

Falyn Hunter Morningstar and Ian Morris

*The paradox of trauma is that it has both the power to destroy
and the power to transform and resurrect.*

~ Peter Levine

MY STORY

Enveloped in the luxurious depths of a deep red leather couch, a soft
dolphin blanket cocooned my weary body. My head nestled on a pillow
that whispered of simpler times. As my gaze drifted, the confines of the
kingdom faded away, replaced by a boundless wilderness where I roamed
free alongside my trusty companions, Timon and Pumbaa.

"Hakuna matata," I murmured. No worries. A carefree mantra,
a balm for the pressures of life and the secrets I bore. Languid paws
dangling, I peered skyward at the stars, certain that a *greater force* was
guiding me. This higher force will visit again, but for now, this respite
from responsibility held me captive.

"Falyn, I'm home." My mother's voice pierced the tranquility, drawing
me back to the present moment.

"Hey Mom, okay," I replied.

"You're still in your pajamas. Have you been watching movies all day? Is that The Lion King movie?" Her concern hung in the air, palpable.

"Yeah, I'm just tired," I responded, acutely aware of the hours that melted away in the screen's flickering light. The realization of my prolonged inactivity washed over me, accompanied by a sudden pressing need to relieve myself.

My gosh, it's almost five p.m. Didn't I disappear at nine this morning?

As I moved to stand, a sharp hiss escaped my lips. The discomfort was no longer a secret; it had grown into a persistent ache, demanding to be acknowledged and voiced.

My mind swirled with worry. It was time to divulge the truth to my mother, no matter how difficult the words may be. After all, secrets have a way of festering, much like the pain that now accompanied my every step.

Alright, let's pause for a moment. This story stirs some emotions, and I find myself tearing up. To ground myself, I'm pressing my feet into this acupressure pillow, centering myself in the present moment. Let me give you some context before we delve deeper into this memory.

I was eight years old during this scene, and it was summer break. Although my parents sometimes left me home alone, my dad worked for himself and was often in and out of the house gathering supplies. So, I was never truly alone. At times, my grandparents stepped in to watch over my older brother and me. He was a bundle of energy, bouncing from one thing to another, demanding their attention. Meanwhile, I was content with one thing.

I want to make it clear that I'm incredibly grateful for my family and the extraordinary life they gave me. However, there were still some events that happened beyond their control, which they couldn't predict or shield me from. It's interesting how everyone processes things differently—food, social cues, emotions, and life itself.

Growing up, I was quite shy and seemed to be attached to something, whether it was a book, stuffed animal, or computer. In fact, my mom has an old photograph of me sitting on a plastic swirly chair, engrossed in a boxy computer. She said, "You were always a curious child learning something." It was like I could "disappear" into these activities, seeking refuge from reality.

This ability to transport myself into different worlds eventually led me to recognize some painful signs, which we'll revisit now.

"Mom," I began, my voice trembling, "there's something I need to tell you." The tension in my throat felt like an uninvited guest—a stubborn frog nestled deep within my windpipe, constricting my voice and leaving me trapped between the desire to speak my truth and the fear of judgment that kept me mute.

She turned away from the refrigerator door, her concern evident in the lines of her face. "Of course, sweetie. What's wrong?"

Taking a breath to steady myself, I fought against the rising tide of emotion. Despite my efforts, tears welled in my eyes as I struggled to put my feelings into words. Summoning the courage, I began, "I don't know what to do. Something is wrong, and it's hurting down there." My voice wavered as I grappled with the anxiety that accompanied me.

Sensing my distress, my mom knelt beside me, one knee resting on the floor, and gently placed her hands on my arms. I was hunched over, sobbing with my hands shielding my eyes, trying to hide from the overwhelming pain and embarrassment.

Gently, she inquired, "Is it hurting all the time, or just when you pee?"

As I fought back tears and sniffled to clear my nose, "it hurts every time I even hold my pee for just a little bit," I managed to say through my sobs, "and it's only getting worse."

My mom embraced me tightly, reassuringly saying, "It's going to be alright, sweetie. We'll get this checked out, and I'm here for you every step of the way."

We arrived at the hospital since urgent care centers were yet to be commonplace. We were relieved to find my father already there, waiting. Upon our arrival, the staff quickly ushered me into a room. The details of this part remain blurry in my memory, but the fear I felt was unmistakable.

The procedure provoked an onslaught of unbearable pain, prompting a chorus of agonized cries that echoed through the halls.

"Oww! Eek!" I wailed, my voice trembling with distress.

The intensity of my anguish was such that my father could hear my whimpers from the waiting room. Even now, the memory brings a prickle of tears to my eyes.

The ensuing bladder infection was both physically and emotionally distressing. The invasive flushing procedure, involving the insertion of a tube into my urethra, felt far from gentle, leaving me with a lingering sense of vulnerability and violation. That moment remains etched in my memory, contributing to a deep-seated mistrust of doctors who lack compassion. It's worth noting that the infection was caused by a combination of factors: habitual bladder-holding, inadequate wiping techniques, and incomplete bladder emptying.

The disconnection of sensation from my bladder led to even more disconnection from my power source—the sacredness of my womb. The connection between my brain and my ovaries became nonexistent soon after my 16th birthday when I started the birth control pill. The male bodies I let in my space, disrespecting myself further, displayed the disconnect. You know that *greater force* I felt guiding me earlier, but ignored? I hadn't heard it for many years.

The impact of neglecting my body at such a young age—just eight years old—was significant and far-reaching. It was but one instance among many, yet I've come to recognize my body's profound wisdom. Amidst the pain and confusion, my body fiercely attempted to protect me, and for that, I'm deeply grateful. With a newfound appreciation, I now see my body as the beautiful, intricate masterpiece it truly is.

How did I get to this perspective? I'm so excited to share this with you!

Energy encompasses more than physical exertion; it's the unseen, yet ever-present force of pulsating frequencies that permeate every aspect of our existence, uniting us with the world around us in an intricate, harmonious web. Every element carries its own distinct energy, or frequency. Everything is "in relationship."

- The food you eat holds a certain quality. Higher-quality items, such as fresh, organic produce or meat from a farmers' market, resonate at a higher frequency. This higher frequency uplifts your body, keeping your organs, enzymes, and tissues functioning optimally.

- Your everyday devices—cell phones, routers, and those hard-to-spot 5G towers—radiate frequencies that affect your body.

- The act of watching the sunrise, soaking in its rays with your naked eyes, exposes you to a unique frequency that can influence your own.

- Your interactions with others, whether intimate or casual, carry their own energetic signatures. When someone is in a bad mood, you may find yourself feeling the same. This is the power of frequency at work.

- Even the music you hear in everyday settings—on the radio or at the grocery store—has a frequency that intermingles with your conscious and unconscious self.

Remember, everything you encounter, from the food you consume and the gadgets you rely upon to the emotions you experience, resonates with a distinct frequency. It's the heartbeat of life itself.

Without conscious awareness and deliberate intention, the types of energy that surround us can inadvertently cause misalignment.

In my own life, I coped with feeling unsafe by retreating inward, detaching from my physical self. This disconnection was exacerbated by an environment characterized by an unhealthy diet, exposure to negative media, harmful language, secondhand smoke, negative human energy, and suppressed emotions. For a sensitive individual like myself, these "little" influences carried significant weight in shaping my frequency.

At a crucial juncture, the urgency to reconnect became paramount, as my very health hung in the balance. The powerful *greater force* that had long *kind of* guided me now demanded attention, compelling me to navigate this path of rediscovery. As an independent adult, I recognized the responsibility to stay curious and untangle this complex web rested solely on my shoulders.

Faced with the urgent questions of why my body seemed to be failing me and what crucial piece I was missing, I immersed myself in the world of wellness, determined to uncover the answers that would guide me toward healing and balance.

My exploration encompassed:

- Comprehensive functional lab tests to identify underlying physical concerns such as gut distress and hormone imbalances.

- A functional medicine certification that was not only about understanding the body's interconnected systems, but also about becoming a practitioner capable of helping others.

- Absorbing wisdom from personal development resources, emphasizing the power of mindset on well-being.

- Opening myself to guided meditation, beginning with five minutes a day, and incorporating intentionally curated music to cultivate my own serene frequency.

- Adopting natural supplements and tailored protocols to guide my body back to its optimal state.

- Collaborating with trauma-informed specialists and undertaking self-experimentation, and introspection, to forge an emotional connection with my body's unspoken stories.

- Surrounding myself with a nurturing environment that fostered growth and encouragement.

Through years of dedication and self-discovery, I honed my ability to discern the subtle messages my body conveys and to perceive the energies that envelop me. Embracing my heightened sensitivity, I transformed what was once a source of vulnerability into a gift—one that has empowered me to reshape my world and frequency.

The transformative journey I embarked upon ultimately led me to a serendipitous encounter with an extraordinary individual, Ian Morris. Little did I know that the popular Paul Chek podcast, in which Ian shared his captivating story, mission, and triumphs, would pave the way for a profound connection, both in life and in business. The divine intervention that brought us together remains a source of awe and wonder. Let me gracefully craft these next *two paragraphs* before I dive into Ian. I'm so excited for you to get to know a little bit about this amazing human.

A virtuoso with over 20 instruments at his command, Ian is the visionary behind Frequency Minded Music™ (FMM) and the LTS Method with the company Listening to Smile. These remarkable innovations have made a huge impact across diverse populations and borders. His groundbreaking work has benefited veterans' organizations, cancer institutes, individuals with disabilities, hospice care facilities, and numerous holistic practitioners spanning over 14 countries, showcasing the boundless potential of his creations to foster healing and harmony using FMM.

The fateful encounter with Ian opened new doors of personal growth, catalyzing a profound metamorphosis in my self-expression, heart, womb space, and the practical application of our teachings, both together and separately. Our collaboration has been an absolute joy, resulting in the creation of vocal-guided meditation albums that have deepened my understanding and connection to frequency, while also expanding our businesses significantly.

Okay, phew. End of the *two paragraphs*. Dear readers, prepare to be captivated by the extraordinary journey of a man whose life could inspire an entire movie series. Ian's story is one of resilience, unwavering commitment to personal growth, and an innate ability to transform adversity into opportunity.

To merely scratch the surface, from an early age, Ian faced challenges in the form of dyslexia, which made the traditional learning model an arduous climb. However, instead of allowing these obstacles to deter him, Ian chose to forge his path by seeking alternative learning methods that embraced his natural talents and creativity.

Throughout his life, Ian experienced a series of profound losses that deeply impacted him. Losing 14 loved ones tested his strength and resilience, as he held his grief close to his heart, often prioritizing the well-being of others over his processing. This emotional weight began to take its toll, leaving Ian searching for a way to transform his pain into purpose and support others who were navigating their own struggles.

In late 2012 and early 2013, Ian received a life-changing colon cancer diagnosis. This pivotal moment became a catalyst for his profound exploration into the realms of healing frequencies, nutrition, and deep emotional work. As Ian delved deeper into these holistic approaches, he was able to heal himself naturally over the next year and a half. Later, in 2017, he applied his knowledge and experience to help his mother heal naturally from breast cancer.

Ian's understanding of the interconnectedness of music, art, and well-being has revolutionized these industries in unprecedented ways. Over the past decade, he has consistently produced an album every single month that integrates intentionality through astrology, human design, and channeling. This is how FMM came to be what it is today. This music sets itself apart from the entertainment-based music industry, as it focuses on healing, release work, and the movement of stagnant energy.

The distinguishing factor that makes FMM powerful is the variety of frequencies and genres it includes. Ian incorporates chakra frequencies in three tunings, body organ frequencies, planetary frequencies, and enhanced binaural beats. Genres are all across the board from hip hop, to spa music, yoga, electronic, traditional deep meditation tracks, to lofi hip hop, shamanic drumming, and much more. These diverse styles serve to empower every single listener's taste in their individual healing journeys and truly help their *nervous system regulate* better in the chaotic world.

Furthermore, Ian's innovative approach to music extends beyond the creation process. He has developed a music licensing program that not only safeguards the intellectual property of artists, but also allows business owners to generate revenue in a previously untapped manner. This pioneering program demonstrates Ian's dedication to fostering a supportive environment within the industry so everyone wins and we all stay in integrity.

To be frank, even after my functional medicine certification, I knew there was still a crucial element missing: *nervous system regulation*. While supplements, diet, and exercise play a role in overall wellness, they can't foster the same transformative shift that arises from cultivating a balanced nervous system. This realization laid the foundation for the creation of the Radiant Balance System™—a comprehensive approach to wellness that harmonizes these various elements of nutrition, sonic, movement, somatic release, lab testing, and natural supplementation for optimal well-being.

Ian and I embody the mindset of lifelong learners, always open to new ideas and methods. We believe that there is never just one path to healing, and we are committed to empowering others by sharing tools and techniques that have worked for us. By encouraging people to embrace what resonates with them, Ian and I nurture a supportive and transformative environment for individuals seeking personal and collective healing.

The point in this entire chapter is to enhance your frequency while transmuting and letting go of the frequencies that aren't harmonious. The subtleties of making space within your nervous system are massively influential to your health and well-being.

THE TOOL

It's time to learn just one tool to feel more open and safer within. Life can be hectic, making it tough to find space for growth, love, and self-reflection. Get ready to embark on a somatic journey with "The Heart's Essence," a Frequency Minded Music™ track by Listening to Smile.

1. Grab your phone or computer, plus headphones, and visit the link at the end of this chapter. Press play and let "The Heart's Essence" envelop you.

2. Get cozy in your favorite chair, with your feet grounded and your posture tall. As the music begins, inhale deeply through your nose, filling your belly. Slowly exhale through your mouth, releasing tension. The exhale should be longer than the inhale. Repeat four times, each breath more purposeful. As you get more comfortable, you can go deeper into different forms of advanced breathwork. Embrace the moment.

3. Place your hands at the sides of your chest, palms facing out, and envision an invisible barrier representing something you wish to release or push away. I like to think of a brick wall that represents something that I want to let go of. Gently and very slowly push forward, with as much tension in your arms and hands as comfortably possible, guiding the wall away from you. Maintain steady breathing.

4. With your arms extended, release your shoulder blades, allowing them to spread out and extend your arms even further. Pause. We're creating so much space.

5. Rest your arms on your lap, pause again. Notice any changes within. Your awareness notices the music again. Rest in it.

6. Repeat the arm extension twice more, pausing to observe each time. Yawns, deep breaths, or relief indicate shifts in your nervous system. If you don't experience any changes, it doesn't mean something is off. Perhaps next time you will. The repetition creates familiarity in your nervous system, so downshifting into a calmer state will happen faster.

7. Let the track continue and drift into peaceful meditation, cultivating a sense of safety and space within. Allow "The Heart's Essence" to nurture your reconnection with your inner self.

Stay curious. It's the moment-by-moment awareness that makes this life a gift.

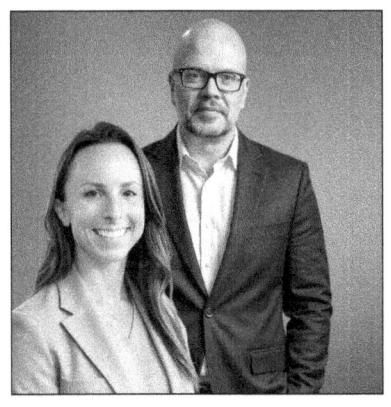

Falyn Hunter Morningstar and **Ian Morris** are visionary entrepreneurs whose curiosity continues to transcend boundaries in the pursuit of global wellness. As influential leaders in the industry, they are reshaping how we approach health and well-being. Falyn's innovative Radiant Balance System™ seamlessly melds mindful healing with Functional Diagnostic Nutrition®, emphasizing movement, nutrition, emotional regulation with sonic and somatic releases, and laboratory testing for optimal well-being.

The duo's partnership extends to Listening to Smile, a music therapy company co-founded by Falyn and Ian. Ian, a gifted sound alchemist, crafts transformative Frequency Minded Music™ tracks every month, and together they design immersive experiences and certifications for clients, organizations, and event groups. Drawing upon their expertise in somatic practices, meditation, and sonic therapies, they cultivate profound transformation opportunities.

What sets Falyn and Ian apart is their dedication to bridging clinical and integrative medicine, with mindfulness, frequency, and somatic communities. Their synchronized approach weaves the wellness and sonic landscapes, inviting us all to step into a brighter, more balanced future.

Connect with Falyn and Ian: https://1qr.com/falynandian

CHAPTER 20

Curiosity Saved This Pussy Cat

It's Your Turn to Save Your Own Life

Natalie V. Petersen

*There is more wisdom in your body
than in your deepest philosophy.*

~ Friedrich Nietzsche

MY STORY

Where I come from, emotions were a considerable liability.

As an example, there was a sense of gratitude among many in my family for those of us who came with regular periods, because that allowed everyone to prepare for whatever storm was sure to arrive.

All of the women in my family were emotional. Both sides. Doomed.

No, we didn't actually talk about all of this outright. This was the 70s, 80s, and early 90s.

In my house, though, my dad kept a calendar on the fridge with deep, red, Bic-penned lines drawn from one corner diagonal to the other:

X X X X X X X

X's on each of the seven (six, if we were lucky) days, every 27.5 days, for the year ahead, for everyone's information. My mom's 'time of the month' was something we always knew was coming. And the last X seemed to represent a sigh of relief.

"You're welcome," this handy display seemed to say.

For most of my adult life, this bit of my childhood and young adulthood memories enraged me, downright offended the woman in me. I wasn't able to put words around it that weren't loaded and meant to *ZING!* across your awareness, but I sourced much of my contorted sense of womanhood to this calendar, this annual customer appreciation freebie from our local Pine River Valley Bank.

Not the promotional item, no.

But the Rocky Mountain seasonally-landscaped backdrops to misogyny, ignorance, emotional manipulation, and internalized patriarchy—served with a side of shame tactics and control?

Ya, that would be IT.

Emotions? I learned one solution. *You're female and likely broken. Medicate.*

"This is just the way it is, Natalie," I was often told by my mom or grandmothers when I asked about women-oriented anything. My sweet mom was on medication until her last breath, long ago accepting that, despite my argument on countless occasions, she was 'just broken.'

I was taught overtly and through unconscious biases rooted generations deep: *the female body, females in business, females in government, females at home, and females as they relate to men are inferior and weak. Our bodies are different, soft, and predictably unpredictable.*

I learned what a Lady is from my ridiculously creative and coiffed Southern belle Grandma Sue. How do *you* do?

And I learned what a good corporate Housewife is from my Rocky Mountain-high, closet actress, Grandma Natalie.

Ugh, I learned what a Whore is from my mom after she read my diary in 5th grade and misunderstood a simple first kiss to be an act of sliding down a very steep and slick slope to evil darkness, as especially evidenced by the dark eyeliner and bright blue mascara I was testing out. I was flirting with deadly sins and eternal Hell.

I was too interested in makeup, more than enough for many people already. In her near-perfect cursive and eloquent, English-teacher way, my mother's letter left for me amidst my stuffed animals, my diary open to the pages of my indiscretions staged neatly on the side, she shared what she thought was best. My translation, nearly four decades later, is:

> *Tuck in, read the room, men are going to misunderstand and*
> *try to have sex with you, and that is only allowed for your*
> *husband. You are saving yourself for him only. Help where*
> *you're necessary, even and especially where it's not obvious*
> *and might be construed as anything other than perfect.*
> *This is the gift and curse of being female.*

"But WAIT! That does NOT sound FAIR! None of this does! It contradicts what you told me yesterday! And the day before!" I'd exclaim in my own confused, theatrical ways.

We weren't to talk about what felt like an imbalance between us, men and women, nope. And no matter your gender, if we had a mouth, we would be tolerated, to a point.

Without looking too close at the interwoven origin stories, you'll see substance, physical, and emotional abuse threaded through every branch of my family tree. Grandma Sue, Grandma Natalie, and my mother, Suzette, were married to men with substance abuse issues, and all three of them were daughters of fathers with the same. They all endured physical and emotional injuries throughout their married lives.

Just as sadly, the men in the equation were all sons of fathers or mothers or both parents with substance, physical, and emotional abuse in their homes. Their brave stories break my heart, too.

All of these wildly beautiful humans, each of whom came honestly into their own way of understanding and surviving in this world, were the first to teach me how to be human. More specifically, they molded me to be what I reflect now on as a white, heterosexual, God-fearing, baby-making, emotionally- and sexually-stunted, people-pleasing, driven (but not too and politely so), as close-to-perfect as she can get without offending anyone, definitely-but-not-too-much, American female.

With this as the ecosystem in which I was being reared, I learned very early in my life to forage for information to help me understand the gaps in what I saw and what I knew in my heart to be my Truth.

I learned early to ask questions. And I loved listening to the answers.

Do not for a minute hear me saying my young life wasn't ridiculously and poetically happy. It was, and I have hours upon hours of tales and adventures, lessons of love and wild, feral living in the high elevations of Southwest Colorado and by the riverside of Los Pinos in my hometown of Bayfield.

Our foundation, however, the bedrock of our little family, was built on a grand concoction of thinking pulled from the likes of the pages of the King James version of the Holy Bible, Dr. Benjamin Spock's *Baby and Child Care*, and James Dobson's *Dare to Discipline*.

> *"21 Submitting yourselves one to another in the fear of God.*
> *22 Wives, submit yourselves unto your own husbands, as unto the Lord. For the husband is the head of the wife, even as Christ is the head of the church: and he is the savior of the body.*
> *[...]*
> *33 Nevertheless, let every one of you in particular so love his wife even as himself; and the wife see [sic] that she reverence her [sic] husband."*

~ Ephesians 6: Concerning the duties of wives

> *"An adolescent girl is much less often overawed by her mother than a boy is by his father, so her rivalrousness is more apt to be expressed openly around the house, not often in academic failure. A girl can even be flirtatious with her father right under her mother's nose or reproach her mother for not being nice enough to her father. Few boys would dare to taunt their father in such ways."*

~ Dr. Spock on Puberty Development, Physical Changes, 584.
Rivalry with parents.

"Pain is a marvelous purifier...It is not necessary to beat the child into submission; a little bit of pain goes a long way for a young child. However, the spanking should be of sufficient magnitude to cause the child to cry genuinely."

~ *From Dare to Discipline,* by James Dobson

So, I present to you today a born-again human who had to tackle some pretty significant misunderstandings about how this living thing works. The -isms I can sling alone will make you dizzy, and you'd be right to wonder if I'm still confused, or at least pretty rattled and maybe irritated.

I'm not. Through diligent, oftentimes brutal excavation of my insides in search of anything out of alignment with my soul, I released myself from the binds of the conditioning of the generations before me.

I release myself anew every day so that I might forge my own path, my own Truth, not someone else's.

No one's but my own.

My mission on the planet that I've been blessed to come to know is to weave new stories that dance with and unwind and inform and allow my extended soul family, that's you and you and you, unconditionally, to find present-tense purpose. My father and mother, their mothers and fathers, and those mothers and fathers and humans before them, were glorious beings with purpose, too, and in *their* present tense, what they did made sense.

Living free of these binds, releasing the expectations and circumstances that created them, doesn't mean I disown my family. I embrace them. It is a commitment to my Truth first that I understand and love these deep, dense, and complex roots of my existence, every one of them.

Finding this alignment in my Truth took work, some of it pretty gnarly, as you can imagine given the buzzwords and keywords I can drop like a rap song. However, as I chipped away at my origin story and set up timelines of a-ha's and infractions to spirit, I dug into the sludge of my deep, dark shadows surrounding my understanding of my Self, my body, and my faith.

Addiction, mental illness, suicide, emotional abuse, racism, sexism, misogyny, narcissism—to find my Spirit, the one writing this to you now, I had to get curious.

I had to quit worrying about the outside's opinion of me, especially those folks who reared me! I had to trust that we would all get back on the same page eventually, if even by a roundabout way that left all of us with our own scars and still-unanswered questions.

Today, writing is an expression of my soul-level work in real time, and I'm called to share my journey and make introductions to the people from whom I've learned, not out of cockiness, but confidence. Confidence that my courage will resonate with you in some way, if even just a tickle. And that, as I like to say, you'll make one nudge, take one step forward in your favor.

THE TOOL

Yep, you guessed it, and you can't be surprised.

As a human, you're bestowed with the universally accepted, irrevocable license to be curious.

But, I want to encourage you to consider a few modifications to the light-and-fluffy kind of curiosity.

This is not "Ooh, what's that over there?" curiosity.

This is a sacred, gritty kind of curiosity that refuses to accept "This is just how it is" as an answer.

The kind that burns through shame, inherited trauma, and religious gaslighting.

The kind that dares to ask anyway—even when it gets you labeled as too much, too loud, too rebellious, too sexual, too emotional, too female, too "other"!

Your tool is the kind of curiosity necessary to save your spirit. The kind that turns survival into sovereignty.

CURIOSITY

This isn't just an inquisitive thought. This is a full-body, Spirit-led, soul-disrupting tool for transformation. It got me asking the questions no one dared to say out loud. It cracked open the shame. It brought me face to face with the stories that weren't mine—and gave me the courage to write new ones of my own.

Now it's your turn.

Start here:

- What part of your story still doesn't make sense, and who told you to stop asking?
- Whose voices live in your head, and how many are actually yours?
- Where do you feel fragmented—and what might happen if you let yourself want to be whole?
- Who around you actually sees you? Not your performance. You.
- And this one: Who would you *be* if you didn't believe you were broken?

Let curiosity be your flashlight. Your crowbar. Your prayer.

Ask the questions. Follow the nudges. Interrupt the cycles.

And understand. This isn't a solo mission. Mental and spiritual health is an all-body, all-community issue. We heal together all the time, always in motion—or not at all.

This isn't about striving. This is about remembering. Returning. Reclaiming.

Being curious about your own well-being—and the people who *want* to support it—is an act of self-respect and self-love. And you don't have to earn that love. It's already yours.

Who in your circle is safe enough to think out loud with? (Hint: not everyone.)

What tools are already right in front of you that you've been too busy, too burdened, or too burned to notice?

Keep it simple. Write them down. Circle them. Try one.

And if you don't know where to start, or everything feels too tangled to even begin, hear this:

You don't have to do it alone.

If all else fails? Reach out. I mean it.

I call myself an accomplice on purpose.

Because when you're ready, I'm already here.

Try me! Try any of my co-authors you find with me here!

And just in case, accept this bonus tool as an easy and private way to begin to dabble in what it means to be curious about your life. You can download it and join the movement of other Healing-Curious Humans at https://1qr.com/healingcurioushumans.

THE WHEEL OF WELLBEING

On a clean piece of paper, draw a large circle that takes up much of the page. Divide the circle into quarters. Then divide each of those in half again. You should have eight total sections in the circle.

In this model, there are eight categories of wellbeing you can consider. Name each line as follows:

1. Emotional
2. Occupational
3. Environmental
4. Financial
5. Intellectual
6. Spiritual
7. Social
8. Physical

You can rename these lines to be more applicable to your life. The point is to take inventory of the most important areas of your wellbeing, those areas of your life that make you whole as a human.

Plot your current satisfaction with each category on each line, with 1 being 'very dissatisfied' in the middle of the circle where all categories meet, and 10 being 'fully satisfied' on the outer edge.

Draw a line connecting the dots when you are done.

What do you observe about the shape? If you rearrange categories/sections, does the shape change? Based on the results, to which area of your life are you immediately drawn?

Your next step is to free-write words and phrases, make drawings and doodles, as you think about each key area of your life. Again, being completely honest and assured there is no right or wrong answer in any of this!

And finally, choose one or two areas you'll focus on with a mentor or coach, loved one, or friend, or on your own. You don't have to choose the areas with the lowest satisfaction first. Choose the ones you want to improve the most or the ones that will help strengthen your sense of identity.

Remember, the complete worksheet will guide you through this process, helping you create a wheel of wellbeing that you can reflect on as you go.

I love you. Unconditionally so.

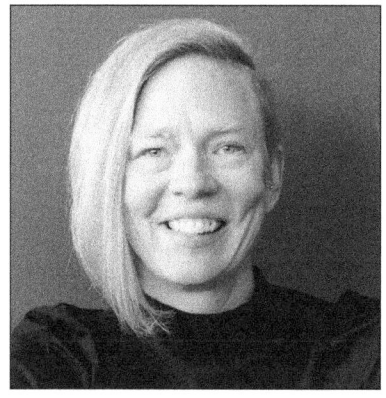

Natalie V. Petersen, or Natalie P. to friends, is a communications strategist, bestselling author, speaker, podcast host, and spiritual misfit and mentor with a rebellious heart and a reverent soul. She's the creator of *Healing-Curious Humans*, a growing movement that explores the wide-open landscape of personal transformation, non-religious spiritual practices, and radical self-reclamation.

With a background spanning media, marketing, storytelling, and mental health advocacy, Natalie has spent 25+ years helping people name their truth, own their voice, and live lives that actually fit. Her work lives at the intersection of identity, expression, and soul-level alignment.

She doesn't teach from a pedestal—she walks beside you as an accomplice. Natalie believes that healing doesn't happen in a vacuum and that wholeness is a community project. Her own story is a fierce and tender reckoning with generational conditioning, religious programming, mental health cycles, and what it means to live fully awake in a world that prefers you asleep.

Through *Healing-Curious Humans*, her signature mentorship offerings, and her unfiltered podcast, *Think Out Loud with Me*, Natalie creates brave, irreverent, loving spaces for people to get curious, get honest, and get free. Whether she's guiding you through the Wheel of Wellbeing, handing you a microphone, or helping you rewrite your origin story, her work is rooted in one thing: **we are not broken—we are becoming**.

She currently lives in Loveland, Colorado, where she's raising kids, goofing off with her sweetheart, building weird sacred shit, and calling in a new kind of leadership: human-first, Spirit-led, and wildly alive.

Connect with Natalie:

https://www.1qr.com/nataliep

Acknowledgements

BEING HUMAN TAKES COURAGE.

To fully actualize our potential, it's easy to believe we need to force our way there. But more often, it's in the surrender—in relinquishing control—that we recover our original intention for arriving in this life, in this time, among this wild, beautiful, thrilling, often overwhelming world of other beings.

I want to acknowledge the human in each of us who wakes up in a state of *what if?* This little, bitty blip of a curious thought led you here to this very moment together.

That is so stinkin' badass. Right?!?

And then? Well, then there are the storytellers in this first volume of *Stories, Tools + Community for Healing-Curious Humans*, who are some of the most fascinating souls I've ever met. I honor each of them for the compassion and commitment they showed throughout this journey— for birthing their truth, for making space for the emotions of "not enough" and "not worthy," and for choosing to show up for themselves and for strangers who became lifelong friends. This book is not just a collaboration—it is communion, and you all partook in life-changing work with me.

Thank you for trusting me. Together, we went between the lines, deep into uncharted territory, and discovered treasures of our life stories to alchemize in real-time for others. Let our brave words be received as they are intended: a gift of **unconditional love**.

I also want to express my heartfelt thanks to Laura Di Franco and the Brave Healer Productions team. Laura, you are a partner in life and in art. I believe in you, sister.

To the mentors and teachers who shaped me in ways you may never fully know, but I hope I have tried to impress, thank you, too.

Thank you, each of you, for witnessing my becoming—and for standing so fiercely in your own. Especially Andi Burgis and Dr. Ann Gill—your spirits live on in mine. I carry you always.

Lastly, hooray!

To my family—both original and chosen through careful selection while belly-crawling across the valleys and mountains of this miracle of human experience, weaving our lives together forever and ever, amen. Cody, Haylie, Hannah, Paul, Nancy, my whole wild crew of misfit friends, angels, ancestors, squiggly-wigglies, furries, scalies, leafy, dry, and especially those flying high—you are the ones who keep hold of the string tethered to this helium-filled bright balloon of a life I lead with unapologetic abandon. You are my tether, my lift, and my landing. Thank you for loving me in all my attitudes and altitudes.

You keep me sane, grounded, and free.

I love you,

Natalie P.

#healingcurioushumans #thinkoutloudwithme #bedohave #noassholes #loveismyalgorithm #bloomstruck #fromseedtobloom #sonicmeditation

Resources

Given the ever-changing landscape of our everyday life, it is always best to begin a search for your best resources by talking to a trusted source like a family member, close friend, or health professional. As of the publication date, the following resources have been verified as available.

988 Suicide & Crisis Lifeline:

Call or text 988 to connect with trained counselors who can provide support during a crisis. This service is available 24/7, free, and confidential.

SAMHSA National Helpline:

1-800-662-HELP (4357) offers confidential support, information, and referrals for mental health and substance use disorders.

NAMI (National Alliance on Mental Illness):

1-800-950-NAMI (6264) offers information, support, and resources for individuals and families affected by mental illness. NAMI also provides support groups, education programs, and advocacy.

Veterans Crisis Line:

Call 988, then press 1 or text 838255 to connect with the Veterans Crisis Line.

State and Local Resources:

Using any browser and any search engine, look up "local mental health services." Check the websites of your state, county, and local government for information about mental health services in your area. Local Better Business Bureaus have contact information for area non-profits and for-profits that have been validated using a code of ethics.

Youth Resources:

If you're a young human, consider the resources around you carefully. Your family, trusted friends, and your close community are all first points of contact. You can also check your school's health center or counseling services for support, or you can call any of the numbers above. Mental Health America offers a list of resources here: https://mhanational.org/youth-mental-health/kids-and-teens/

www.ingramcontent.com/pod-product-compliance
Lightning Source LLC
Chambersburg PA
CBHW061728120626
46550CB00005B/1743